GET A GRIP ON ARTHRITIS
and Other Inflammatory Disorders

GET A GRIP ON ARTHRITIS
and Other Inflammatory Disorders

Lorna R. Vanderhaeghe

Bearing Marketing Communications
Toronto

First published in Canada in 2004 by
Bearing Marketing Communications Ltd.

2 3 4 5   QCE   08 07 06 05

ISBN: 0-9731803-4-X

Cover by Thrillworks Inc.
Interior book design by BbM Graphics
Edited by Susan Girvan

DISCLAIMER: While all care is taken with the accuracy of the
facts and procedures in this book, the author accepts neither
liability nor responsibility to any person with respect to loss,
injury or damage caused, or alleged to be caused directly or
indirectly, by the information contained in this book. The
purpose of this book is to educate and inform. For medical
advice you should seek the individual, personal advice and
services of a health care professional.

Those wishing to obtain additional copies of this book or
requesting permission to reproduce material from it may contact:

Bearing Marketing Communications Ltd.
5080 Timberlea Blvd., Unit 1
Mississauga, ON
L4M 2W7
905 238 5876

Printed and bound in Canada

CONTENTS

The Inflammation Connection

Common Inflammatory Conditions

Preface

More and more information is accumulating that indicates inflammation plays a major role in the development of many diseases – from arthritis and Alzheimer's disease to heart disease, psoriasis and even stroke. That is because inflammation represents a very basic response by the body to alterations in the cellular environment, whether the cells line the gums (gingivitis), skin (sunburn), arteries (atherosclerosis) or joints (arthritis). The body's most basic purpose for inflammation to repair itself, as well as defend against clear and present dangers.

While the inflammation associated with arthritis or psoriasis is usually quite obvious, the inflammation of most concern in modern life often goes unnoticed. It is the low-grade, chronic inflammation that triggers hardening of the arteries (atherosclerosis), Alzheimer's disease and cancer and that threatens most people's real quality of life. This message is woven throughout Lorna Vanderhaeghe's excellent review of inflammation and how to deal with it through natural, drug-free measures.

In regards to arthritis, whether it is osteoarthritis, gout or rheumatoid arthritis, there is mounting evidence that current medical treatment may be doing more harm than good. The primary drugs used in the treatment of both osteoarthritis and rheumatoid arthritis are the so-called "nonsteroidal anti-inflammatory drugs" or NSAIDs, which include aspirin. Although these drugs are extremely popular, research is indicating that in the treatment of osteoarthritis and rheumatoid arthritis these drugs may be producing short-term benefit, but actually accelerating the progression of the joint destruction and causing more problems down the road. Results of numerous studies have raised some interesting questions: Does medical intervention in some way promote disease progression? Can nutrition and various natural therapies enhance the body's response towards health? The answer to both of these questions, as evident by the information presented in this book, is clearly "yes."

In most cases, the natural approach will provide far greater relief because it addresses the underlying disease process. That is particularly true in regards to dealing with chronic inflammation, whether it is in an obvious form like arthritis or the stealth, seemingly unnoticeable form that increases the risk for heart disease, brain degeneration and cancer.

Lorna does an excellent job of providing real solutions to dealing with arthritis and other inflammatory disease. It is my hope that the readers of this book will follow the recommendations given and experience relief from their arthritis or other inflammatory state without the use of drugs or surgery. I also hope that you will share your experiences with others, including physicians, so that even more people can benefit.

Michael T. Murray, N.D.
August 2004

Acknowledgements

There are always special people who help get a book published.
I would like to acknowledge a few of them.

First, thank you to Michael Murray, N.D. for your kindness and
support since I have joined the Natural Factor's science team.
Deane Parkes, my longtime friend and kindred spirit, you continually
provide me with everything I need to be successful. I am grateful to Dean
and Lou Mosca for thinking of me first to do this project. My editor Susan
Girvan, your expertise in making all of my books better is invaluable.
To my children, Crystal, Kevin, Kyle and Caitlyn who endured and
supported me through another summer of book writing
– I am blessed to have each of you.

Special thanks to the pioneers, physicians and scientists in the fields
of immunology, rheumatology and pain management:
without you, this book would not exist.

For all those persons in pain and suffering with arthritis and
inflammatory disorders, this book is dedicated to you.

The Inflammation Connection

Arthritis, gingivitis, heart disease and psoriasis are conditions that affect very different parts of the body, yet they all have something in common: inflammation. What's more, inflammation is now thought to play a role in dozens of other conditions, from allergies, asthma, bowel disease and autoimmune disorders like lupus to macular degeneration and memory loss.

Inflammation in Action

Inflammation is your immune system's first reaction against infection, and it is a very effective one. When a thorn cuts through the skin on your finger, damaging tissue and allowing invaders like bacteria into your body, your immune system goes to work immediately, sending out many different types of specialized cells, each with their own action. Mast cells — specialized immune cells — release histamine, along with other immune messengers known as cytokines, to alert your body to the problem. Histamine increases blood flow to the injured area, promoting redness and swelling. Macrophages (meaning "large eating cells"), found predominantly in connective tissue and the epidermis of the skin, then enter the fray; they also secrete immune messengers, destroy the bacteria and clean up damaged cells. Other immune cells travel to the area, intensifying the battle, and as the area is cleared, more cells arrive to begin the healing process.

The injured area often becomes hot, red, swollen and painful. The heat is produced by the increased blood flow to the injured area. Redness occurs because the battle and repair processes are underway. And the area usually becomes swollen because of all the

1

fluid and immune cells at the site. Pain is often the first indicator of inflammation. It makes you to take notice and stop moving the affected area to prevent further injury. Think about your last sunburn: how your skin was hot to the touch, swollen and painful. Think about how your gums became inflamed when you flossed too aggressively. Or think about your body's response to an insect bite — these are all signs of inflammation that you can see.

Inflammation is an effective way of ensuring that invaders do not enter your body and create havoc, but when it becomes low-grade and chronic, your immune system's army stays revved up and damages healthy tissues in the crossfire. Scientists are realizing that this life-saving process, designed to ward off bacteria, viruses and parasites, creates disease when it's left unchecked. It leads to the painful and damaging inflammation that attacks joints, organs or arteries. *Get a Grip on Arthritis and Other Inflammatory Disorders* will help you find natural relief from the inflammatory process that is causing the pain and destruction associated with so many common diseases and help reverse that damage.

Causes of Chronic Inflammation

Stress, bacteria, viruses, parasites, environmental poisons, certain foods (including sugar), smoking, high blood-insulin levels and obesity are just a few of the factors that promote inflammation. The fact that we are living a lot longer than our ancestors did may also be contributing to inflammation; as we age, our ability to shut off the inflammatory process often weakens.

FOODS THAT CAUSE INFLAMMATION
The foods you choose can either promote or prevent inflammation. Foods containing arachidonic acid, such as eggs, organ

meats (including liver, heart and giblets), beef and dairy products promote inflammation. Through a complicated process the body breaks down arachidonic acid into inflammatory compounds, including the hormones, prostaglandins and leukotrienes that control the mechanisms of inflammation, constrict blood vessels and promote blood clotting.

Overcooked food or foods cooked at high temperatures (including French fries, blackened and/or barbecued foods, fried chicken — high-heat frying or deep-fried foods) incite the inflammatory response because they create advanced glycation end products (AGES), something the body treats as an invader. AGES are produced when a protein is bound to a glucose molecule, resulting in damaged, cross-linked proteins. As the body tries to break these AGES apart, immune cells secrete large amounts of inflammatory cytokines. Many of the diseases that we think of as part of aging are actually caused by this process. Depending on where the AGES occur, the result can be arthritis, heart disease, cataracts, memory loss, wrinkled skin or diabetes complications, to name a few.

What You Can Do
Eat at least six servings of vegetables and one serving of fruit every day. These are foods that have a low rating on the glycemic index — meaning the body takes longer to break them down into blood glucose — and are the best choices for reducing inflammation (see a sample chart of glycemic index ratings below). The standard, high-carbohydrate, low-protein diet we are eating is disrupting our bodies' ability to regulate blood sugar adequately. It forces our bodies to pump out too much insulin in order to reduce abnormally high blood glucose, and our bodies' cells become resistant to insulin's action. In addition, those high blood-glucose levels increase inflammation — foods low on the glycemic index chart calm the inflammatory process.

Eat moderate amounts of free-range, organic chicken and plenty of fish. Do not eat margarine, shortening or highly processed supermarket oils. Avoid all foods containing trans fats. Read labels; if you see "partially hydrogenated" or "hydrogenated," the food contains trans fats, which promote inflammation. Extra virgin olive oil is the safest oil sold in your local grocery store; later you will read more on essential-fatty-acid-rich oils. Avoid processed foods of all types — they should be labeled, "Warning inflammation will occur if you eat this."

Low-Glycemic-Index (GI) Foods: Moderate consumption of foods rated lower on the glycemic index help reduce inflammation, balance blood sugar, lower insulin requirements, reduce body fat, reduce blood pressure, improve immune system function, promote longevity and provide overall, enhanced well-being. These are foods with a rating of 60 or lower on the scale below. (Ratings are comparative, using glucose as the benchmark.) Just think "natural as Mother Nature intended." Choose foods that are whole foods, not processed, without sugar or fake fats, and protein-enriched to keep your blood-glucose levels within a healthy range and inflammation under control.

Food	Glycemic Index (GI) Rating
Glucose	100
Potato, baked	98
Carrots, cooked	92
Cornflakes	92
White rice, instant	91
Honey	74
Bread, white	72
Bagels	72
Melba toast	70
Potato, mashed	70

Food	Glycemic Index (GI) Rating
Bread, wheat	69
Table sugar	65
Beets	64
Raisins	61
Bran muffin	60
Pita	57
Oatmeal, large flake (not instant)	55
Popcorn (air popped)	55
Buckwheat	54
Banana	53
Brown rice	50
Grapefruit juice, unsweetened	48
Bread, whole grain pumpernickel	46
Soy milk	44
Bread, dark whole grain rye	42
Pinto beans	42
Whole grain pasta	41
Apples	39
Tomato juice, canned, unsweetened	38
All-bran cereal	38
Tomatoes	38
Yogurt, plain	38
Yams	37
Chick peas	36
Skim milk	32
Organic strawberries (i.e., pesticide-free)	32
Real egg fettuccini	32
Kidney beans	29
Whole grain spaghetti, protein-enriched	27
Peaches	26
Cherries	24

Food	Glycemic Index (GI) Rating
Non-starchy vegetables: arugula, asparagus, lettuces, chard, broccoli, avocado, eggplant, cucumber, cauliflower, kale, celery, all seed sprouts, Brussels sprouts, zucchini, scallions, rhubarb, purple cabbage, mushrooms	Lower than 20

Meat, poultry, fish, eggs, fats and oils are not rated because they have almost no carbohydrates. This means they are low-GI foods, but remember to avoid red and organ meats and too many eggs because they promote inflammation.

EATING TOO MUCH CAUSES INFLAMMATION

We know that overeating promotes the inflammatory response and suppresses the immune system. Tests performed by the National Institute on Aging revealed that when animals were fed 50 percent fewer calories per day, their immune response improved, the amount of inflammatory cytokines in circulation was reduced, thymus size was maintained and inflammation-fighting T-cell function improved. This study looked at higher and lower calorie consumption; it did not distinguish among the types of calories consumed. Heavy, red-meat-based diets or lots of sugar-laden foods would definitely have a negative impact on immune function and promote inflammation, whereas calories in the form of fruits, vegetables, legumes, nuts and seeds would improve immunity. No matter what the food choices, moderation is the key in terms of both total daily quantity and amounts consumed at one time. Generally, five or six small meals (of the right foods) throughout the day are considered to be healthier than consuming fewer large ones.

FAT CELLS INCREASE INFLAMMATION

It is known that even an extra 20 pounds can create an abundance of inflammation in the human body and lower overall immunity. Weight management is an important aspect of maintaining a balanced immune system and controlling inflammation. With over 50 percent of North Americans overweight, and an additional 15 percent or more classed as obese, public health care planners expect to see a tremendous increase in inflammatory diseases. Fat cells act like immune cells and secrete inflammatory factors (histamines and cytokines), especially during weight gain. The more fat cells you have, the more potential there is for inflammation.

Weight gain also puts tremendous pressure on joints. For every ten pounds of weight gained, 40 pounds or more of additional pressure is put on hips and knees, compressing cartilage and collagen, grinding down bones, promoting damage and the inflammatory response.

POOR SLEEP CAUSES INFLAMMATION

Inflammatory cytokines are secreted at a higher rate by those who have insomnia, compared to those who do not. During sleep, the body regenerates and the immune system calms down. Lack of restorative sleep is a major promoter of inflammation. People with rheumatoid arthritis or other autoimmune disorders know this, because lack of sleep due to pain associated with their condition promotes further flare-ups and more pain.

Up to 33 percent of North Americans are in chronic pain, which disables more people than cancer and heart disease combined. Lost workdays, workers' compensation claims and medical expenses associated with chronic pain are estimated to cost the both Canada and the U.S. over US$100 billion annually. Adequate rest is essential when battling inflammation.

Melatonin, 5-HTP and valerian, among other natural sleep aids, should be used to improve sleep and calm the inflammatory response.

Key Agents of Inflammation and Disease

An immune system running unchecked can promote a variety of debilitating conditions. What can you do to protect yourself from potential damage? What are some of the key immune system messengers that promote inflammation and how do these messengers cause conditions like Alzheimer's, heart disease and more?

All the cells of the immune system send out chemical signals that tell other immune cells where to go and what to do. In order to control or reverse the inflammatory process, we need to control the secretions of some of these chemicals. Throughout the book, you will see references to how the actions of some of the most common, disease-promoting inflammatory immune factors cause certain disorders, and how to stop them in their tracks.

Histamine is a chemical found in many cells of the body but is abundant in the mast cells of connective tissue (muscles, tendons, ligaments and fascia). It is released in response to injury or invasion. It causes the blood vessels to open wide, promoting pain and the runny nose seen in allergic reactions; histamine also increases the permeability of blood vessels.

Interleukin-1 (IL-1) is a cytokine that induces fever or heat in the body. Fever slows down a virus or bacteria. Macrophages, the giant eating cells of the immune system, secrete most of the IL-1. This chemical tells other immune cells to join the fight.

IL-1 is linked to many inflammatory conditions, especially arthritis and Alzheimer's. It also breaks down collagen and connective tissues.

Interleukin-6 (IL-6) is also secreted by macrophages and other immune cells. It tells the immune system to produce antibodies so that if you ever get the same bacteria or virus invading the body again, the immune system will be able to kill it immediately. Abnormal production of IL-6 is associated with autoimmune disorders and allergic conditions. Psoriasis is one condition where IL-6 makes the skin cells reproduce abnormally. IL-6, when in excess, also promotes pain and inflammation and causes certain key cells to make antibodies, called autoantibodies, that can destroy the body's tissues, organs and joints. We see this in those with lupus, Crohn's disease, Type-1 diabetes, rheumatoid arthritis and more. IL-6 also promotes calcium loss from bones, increasing our risk of osteoporosis.

Tumor necrosis factor (TNF) is secreted by macrophages and it induces fever and inflammation.

Antibodies are produced by specialized cells to ensure that when we are exposed to a virus or bacteria a second time, the immune system is ready; some are found in our tears, sweat and saliva. Certain antibodies promote allergic reactions by causing massive amounts of histamine to be released, others coat invaders for destruction, and still other antibodies engulf bacteria.

Prostaglandins are hormone-like, fatty substances (lipids) that are formed when arachidonic acid is broken down. Prostaglandins and inflammation go hand in hand as they promote pain, swelling and redness. Cyclooxygenase, also known as Cox-1 and Cox-2 enzymes, help make prostaglandins. The prostaglandins made by Cox-2 enzymes are inflammatory and make the effects of histamine much worse, increasing the amount of pain experienced. In contrast, Cox-1 enzymes are healing.

C-reactive protein is a substance produced by the liver during an inflammatory response. Dr. Paul Ridker, a cardiologist at Brigham and Women's Hospital, is the scientist who discovered that people who had elevated levels of C-reactive protein (CRP) were at higher risk of heart attack. In fact, those with CRP levels above 3.0 mg/L had a risk of heart attack or stroke three times higher than the risk of those with a reading of less than 0.5 mg/L.

CRP Blood Levels

Ask your physician for a high-sensitivity CRP blood test to discover how inflamed your body is. If you have a CRP level over 3.0 mg/L, you should work to locate the source of inflammation in the body and treat it quickly.

- Optimal: Less than 0.5 mg/L to 1.0 mg/L
- Should be monitored: Between 1.0 mg/L and 3.0 mg/L
- Indicates high levels of inflammation: Over 3.0 mg/L

By monitoring your blood levels of these markers, particularly CRP, you can gauge the level of inflammation in your body and start to take steps to lower or eliminate it. These steps are key in protecting your health — research has linked inflammation to a wide variety of disorders.

INFLAMMATORY AGENTS AND DISEASE
Heart Disease

Heart disease, especially clogged arteries, was thought to be caused by too much LDL (the bad cholesterol) sticking to artery walls. Yet half of those who have a heart attack have normal cholesterol levels. The Physician's Health Study, which looked at CRP levels in 22,000 healthy men and their risk of heart disease, found that there is a direct correlation between inflammation and heart disease. How can this be? In the case of heart disease and inflammation, scientists have learned that, even in those with normal blood cholesterol, occasionally cholesterol finds its way into the lining of the artery and is embedded there as plaque. (Those with high blood cholesterol are at greater risk of this happening.) Macrophages are alerted to the foreign invader and they arrive with other immune cells to eliminate the plaque. These cells bombard the site and the cholesterol plaque is broken away from the artery wall. If the plaque is big enough, it creates a blockage — and a heart attack or stroke.

Women on hormone replacement therapy have to be particularly careful because estrogen (Premarin was used in the studies) increases inflammation in the body and elevates CRP to dangerous levels, indicating a much higher risk of heart attack and, particularly, strokes.

Cancer

High blood levels of CRP also indicate an increased risk of certain cancers. A study published in the *Journal of the American Medical Association* found that those with the highest CRP levels had triple the risk of developing colon cancer when compared to those with the lowest CRP results.

Macular Degeneration

Inflammation is also involved in promoting macular degeneration of the eye, the leading cause of blindness in the elderly. High CRP levels have been found in those who develop the most severe form of macular degeneration.

Type-2 Diabetes

High IL-6 and CRP are good predictors of the development of Type-2 diabetes. Those persons who had the highest blood IL-6 levels had more than double the risk of developing Type-2 diabetes, and those with the highest blood CRP levels had more than four times the risk of Type-2 diabetes, compared to those with low levels of these inflammatory markers.

Alzheimer's Disease

New research shows that an overactive immune system plays a powerful role in causing central nervous system inflammation and destruction of neurons (neurons transmit and receive signals in the brain), promoting memory loss and Alzheimer's disease.

Our brains contain a certain immune cell called a microglia cell, which acts like a macrophage (the "big eater" cells of the immune system of the body). These brain microglia cells release inflammatory immune messengers, including IL-1 and IL-6. Experimental animal studies and clinical trials in humans have shown that these inflammatory immune factors promote the destruction of neurons in Alzheimer's disease brains. In certain animal studies, when IL-1 and IL-6 were blocked, destruction of neurons was halted.

Conventional Treatments for Inflammation

Research is currently underway using drugs to inhibit the inflammatory process, instead of just masking the symptoms. The goal is to control pro-inflammatory immune cytokines like Interleukin-1 (IL-1), Interleukin-6 (IL-6), prostaglandins and histamine, among others. Carl Germano and William Cabot, in their book *Nature's Pain Killers*, state that, "IL-1 is directly responsible for breaking down collagen and other connective tissue, increasing inflammatory prostaglandin production and dilating blood vessels — all actions that create pain. IL-6 is a powerful pro-inflammatory factor that contributes to the symptoms of dozens of inflammatory conditions, including rheumatoid arthritis." Bad prostaglandins also cause pain. They are made from enzymes called Cox enzymes. Cox-2 enzymes generate inflammation that causes pain. The goal in preventing inflammation is to halt or control the release of the immune messengers creating the assault on healthy cells and tissues.

Until recently, the goal of conventional medication for treatment of inflammatory conditions has focussed largely on controlling pain, with mixed results.

PAIN MEDICATION DANGERS

North Americans spend over US$3.9 billion on over-the-counter pain medications. Acetaminophen is the most commonly used painkiller, followed by non-steroidal anti-inflammatory (NSAIDs) such as ibuprofen and finally aspirin. More pain medications are purchased for the control of arthritis symptoms than for any other disorder.

Despite the popularity of the various pain medications, their safety is not guaranteed. Unintentional overdoses of acetaminophen are very common. Patients who are in severe pain may be tempted to take too many tablets. The dosage recommendations must be followed carefully. When taken in higher than recommended doses, acetaminophen causes liver damage, particularly when it is combined with alcohol. Acetaminophen overdose is the leading cause of acute liver failure and causes ten percent of all cases of kidney failure. Most people do not realize that they are mixing a deadly concoction when they combine alcohol (even a couple of drinks) with acetaminophen, but liver toxicity can occur even when taking as little as two extra doses per day, combined with alcoholic beverages.

Long-term use of NSAIDs causes 20,000 deaths in the U.S. annually. In addition, over 120,000 North Americans are hospitalized each year, suffering from the side effects of NSAIDs. Side effects include gastrointestinal complaints (bleeding, nausea and vomiting), liver damage, stomach ulcers, allergic reactions, immune system depression, mental confusion and kidney failure. Adverse drug interactions are common and central nervous system toxicity can occur with some of the NSAIDs. Patients receiving corticosteroids and NSAIDs together have a 15 times greater risk for peptic ulcer disease than those who are receiving no medication. The *New England Journal of Medicine* reported that NSAIDs are the cause of 15 percent of all drug-induced cases of kidney failure.

NSAIDs and Joint Destruction

There is also evidence that NSAIDs are counterproductive when it comes to our joints. A study published in *The Lancet* found that NSAIDs contribute to cartilage destruction. Yes, you read that correctly! NSAIDs can cause joint destruction. I reported years ago on a study that examined 294 hip X-rays, finding that the hip joints of patients taking NSAIDs had greater joint destruction than the hip joints of patients not taking NSAIDs. Now a new animal study published in *The Journal of Bone and Mineral Research* has also shown bone repair problems related to NSAIDs. Researchers at the University of Medicine and Dentistry in New Jersey gave 253 rats with broken bones either Vioxx, Celebrex, Indomethacin or no drug. The rats given Vioxx or Celebrex took more than two months to fully heal, and the new bone that formed had a weakened shell. Some bone experts say the results are so compelling that doctors should explain the risk of taking such drugs when treating bone injuries or in relation to spinal surgery.

In addition to concerns about joint damage, Celebrex, a newer type of NSAIDs touted as much safer than earlier versions, may not, in fact, be so safe. Research performed at the University of Pennsylvania Medical Center has found that Celebrex may increase the risk of heart attack and/or stroke. Celebrex is a sulfa drug, like some antibiotics and oral diabetes drugs, and those with sulfa allergies must avoid it. Sulfa allergies affect five percent of the population.

Celebrex, which is much more expensive than common arthritis drugs, is also no better than earlier NSAIDs in terms of undesirable gastrointestinal side effects. Based on evidence of a large clinical trial, researchers found there is a stronger chance than previously thought for users of Celebrex to develop ulcer problems. The trial compared patients taking Celebrex with patients taking ibuprofen and Voltaren (also known as diclofenac). The results showed that there is, in fact, no difference among the three drugs when it comes to gastrointestinal illness. Many arthritis sufferers taking Celebrex have found that the gastrointestinal problems they had with NSAIDs still occur when taking Celebrex. Dr. Simon Huang, a Vancouver rheumatologist who led local clinical trials on Celebrex, found that "although Celebrex has been found to reduce ulcers in the upper GI tract, the effects on the lower GI tract are unknown." In July 2002 Health Canada issued a warning about Celebrex. Ten deaths and over 70 cases of severe gastrointestinal bleeding have occurred in Canadians taking Celebrex over the last three years

Natural Remedies to Stop Inflammation

Many nutrients halt the action of inflammatory cytokines and prostaglandins without the side effects associated with drugs.

They should be considered as excellent anti-inflammatory agents, including boswellia extracts, Celadrin, curcumin, fish oil and vitamins. General descriptions are included below in alphabetical order; specific recommendations for inflammatory conditions are included in the next section, under "Prescription for Health," in order of importance.

BOSWELLIA

Boswellia, an extract from the *Boswellia serrata* tree, has been extensively studied in humans and found to have several powerful anti-inflammatory effects. It inhibits inflammatory factors and the Cox enzyme pathway and therefore reduces inflammatory prostaglandins. It also acts as an analgesic and may improve circulation to damaged joints and inflamed tissue. In one study, 70 percent of rheumatoid arthritis patients had a reduction in pain and stiffness. To verify this finding, researchers gave 17 of the treatment patients receiving Boswellia the placebo pill instead, and their symptoms returned.

CELADRIN

One of the newest, most effective, natural anti-inflammatory products is Celadrin, a patented blend of special fatty acids. Celadrin is available in capsules, tablets, soft gels or as a cream. Both humans and animals have shown remarkable improvements in terms of reduced pain and swelling, increased range of movement and reduction of inflammatory factors when using Celadrin.

Results of a double-blind, multi-center, placebo-controlled trial (the most scientifically validated type) published in the prestigious *Journal of Rheumatology* found that Celadrin, when taken orally, improved joint and mobility problems. Sixty-four participants between the ages of 37 and 77 were given Celadrin capsules. They were evaluated at the beginning, at 30 days and at the end of the 68-day study. Compared to those given a placebo, participants taking Celadrin had more flexibility, fewer aches, less pain and were able to walk longer distances than the placebo group.

On the anecdotal side, Tony Gwynn, eight-time National League batting title winner, has relied on Celadrin to undo 20 years of baseball damage to his knees, and Danny Milsap, an 84-year-old softball pitching legend, uses Celadrin to keep him in the game. In addition, Derek Boosey, Senior Olympic gold medalist in the triple jump in the 55 to 60 age class, has used oral and topical Celadrin to eliminate knee pain. He has also seen his levels of bad cholesterol fall, while his good cholesterol levels have risen; his CRP level is 0.13 mg/dL.

Celadrin is also currently being researched for the treatment of gingivitis, another common inflammatory disorder. Results are expected in 2005.

Anti-inflammatory Cream

Research on the effectiveness of Celadrin cream performed at the University of Connecticut involved 42 patients with osteoarthritis of the knee. Participants received either Celadrin or a placebo cream applied topically. They were evaluated before application of the cream, 30 minutes after, and then again following a 30-day treatment period during which the cream was applied twice a day, morning and evening. The researchers evaluated physical function, postural sway, pain and range of motion. Test of physical function included a timed assessment of how long it took to get up and go from a chair, stair climbing, muscle strength and endurance, and mobility of the knee. The group receiving Celadrin had outstanding results with reduced pain and stiffness, improved balance and strength and better mobility. What was most exciting was that within 30 minutes of applying Celadrin cream, patients experienced a dramatic improvement in all aspects tested. (No difference in the ability to extend the leg was noted between groups.) Results of this study were published in *The Journal of Rheumatology, August 2002*. Another study using Celadrin cream, performed as an extension of the previous study, confirmed earlier research showing improvement in elbow, wrist and knee mobility and significant reduction in pain.

Those using the oral form of Celadrin and the cream together experienced a much faster improvement in pain, swelling and mobility than those using the cream alone.

Celadrin Cream and Psoriasis: Another double-blind, placebo-controlled study using Celadrin cream for the treatment of psoriasis was performed over a 14-day period. Patients were asked to apply the cream to the affected area twice a day. Initial severity of skin scales, patchiness, redness, dryness, crack and raised skin was recorded. Then, after 7 and 14 days, each patient visited a dermatologist for evaluation of skin improvement. Each patient experienced a two-level improvement based on the 6-point Liker scale (0 = no improvement, 5 = significant improvement). This small pilot study found that those using Celadrin cream experienced measurable improvement in their psoriatic condition. Reports from those using Celadrin have sparked the interest in another area of skin healing. A study is underway that looks at Celadrin's effect in reducing wrinkles in the skin. By calming the skin and halting inflammation — which promotes the effects of aging — we can reduce fine lines and wrinkles.

How Celadrin Works

Celadrin works similar to, but much more dramatically than, the essential fatty acids EPA and DHA from fish oils. Fatty acids provide many vital, beneficial effects for the immune and inflammatory responses of the body. Various fatty acids induce changes in cell membranes and the responsiveness of the membrane to certain immune factors. They also play a role in suppressing inflammatory cell functions, decreasing cartilage breakdown (which triggers cell death) and, like NSAIDs, reduce the inflammatory activities of the Cox-2 enzyme.

The esterified (meaning they are stable and do not react with oxygen) fatty acids present in Celadrin have pronounced anti-inflammatory effects, such as the inhibition of inflammation in endothelial cells (thin cells that line the inside of some body cavities) and decreasing the pro-inflammatory effects of other fatty acids like arachidonic acid. The special fatty acids found in Celadrin have also been shown to reduce the production of the negative immune factor IL-6 and to control the immune factors responsible for inflammation. This alone could explain some effects of Celadrin, such as reduction of pain in joints affected by osteoarthritis. These anti-inflammatory functions are very important in preventing further tissue and joint damage while promoting healing. Additionally, the molecules found in Celadrin may play a role in the lubrication of an affected joint. This action, combined with anti-inflammatory effects, explains some of the significant improvements in mobility and function. Such combined effects would appear to be occurring through the application of Celadrin cream in psoriasis. Also, these special fatty acids have been shown to reduce skin inflammation, while providing a sustained moisturizing effect at the site of psoriasis.

Celadrin also works by inhibiting arachidonic acid, one of the main promoters of the inflammatory cascade of immune factors, by inhibiting 5-lipoxygenase — another mediator of inflammation. It may also alter cellular membranes, protecting them from the action of inflammatory cytokines or reducing the secretion of inflammatory cytokines and CRP.

Is Cetyl Myristoleate the same as Celadrin?

No, Cetyl Myristoleate (CMO) is a single carbon-based, fatty acid ester that has not been scientifically validated. The results of one study on CMO, using a small sample of mice, have not been replicated in a scientific setting. A most recent study published in September of 2002 in *Pharmacological Research* attempted to replicate this study design and protocol and found the injection of a human equivalent level of approximately 24,000 mg daily of CMO did not show a significant difference compared to the placebo group. *The Physician's Desk Reference for Nutritional Supplements* states that there is no credible support for claims that CMO is effective in arthritis.

CHONDROITIN SULPHATE

Chondroitin (pronounced con-*droy*-tin) sulphates are natural body lubricants that provide cartilage with its elasticity and provide protection for bones in contact with one another, another shock absorber. By halting the breakdown of old cartilage and stimulating the production of new cartilage, chondroitin sulphate is an effective treatment for the protection of joints. Like glucosamine sulphate (see below), many studies have confirmed the action of chondroitin. Long-term, placebo-controlled, double-blind studies performed in Europe found that chondroitin sulphate reduced pain, and that damage to cartilage from arthritis was repaired to a significant degree within as little as three months. Again, even after the study subjects stopped taking chondroitin, they experienced lasting effects into the post study evaluation period.

DEHYDROEPIANDROSTERONE (DHEA)

DHEA is reduced in those individuals under stress and particularly in those with autoimmune disorders. Studies show that

DHEA reduces the number of attacking antibodies and therefore helps to control autoimmune disorders. DHEA is often very low in Lupus patients. Research using DHEA in an unusually high dose of 200 milligrams per day reduced the symptoms of Lupus significantly. *Caution: 200 milligrams per day should not be consumed without a physician's guidance. Use of DHEA is also cautioned for those with certain cancers because it may convert into testosterone and/or estrogen in the body.*

DEVIL'S CLAW

At the beginning of the last century, European researchers discovered Devil's claw in Namibia, the former South West Africa. It was used as a folk remedy for the aged until it was proven to have therapeutic benefits in treating arthritic symptoms. Many new studies have confirmed Devil's claw as a potent anti-inflammatory. The active ingredient in Devil's claw, standardized harpagosides, was studied in 50 patients suffering with arthritis; results found that arthritis symptoms and severity of pain were markedly decreased. Controlled clinical research in Europe compared the efficacy of a standard anti-arthritic drug, phenylbutazone, with that of Devil's claw. The results revealed Devil's claw to be more effective in reducing pain and inflammation, without the unpleasant side effects associated with the drug.

ESSENTIAL FATTY ACIDS

Essential fatty acids (EFAs) form the lipid layer of all cells in the body and control the development of the brain, eye and nervous system. They also regulate both good and bad prostaglandins that promote smooth muscle contractions and influence hormones. Omega-3 essential fatty acids are abundant in cold-water fish: herring, mackerel, salmon and tuna; and flaxseed and walnut oils. Omega-6 essential fatty acids are found in supermarket canola, sunflower and safflower oils, as well as in the food supplements evening primrose, borage and black current seed oils.

Omega-6 oils should be further classified as good or bad Omega-6 oils. Those containing Gamma-linolenic Acid (GLA) including evening primrose, borage and black current are good, anti-inflammatory oils, whereas canola, sunflower and safflower, when highly refined or eaten in excess, promote inflammation making them "bad." Our diets are predominantly high in the Omega-6 oils found in highly processed foods such as margarines and supermarket vegetable oils. Processed foods should be eliminated from your diet. Instead add fresh, unrefined foods rich in essential fatty acids. Those with inflammatory and/or autoimmune diseases will be the first to notice how effective this simple diet change can be in the reduction of their symptoms.

Early research has shown that essential fatty acids reduce the level of pain stimulators, and researchers have suggested that EFA supplementation is useful in decreasing the pain associated with osteoarthritis. EFA supplementation can help chronic inflammatory degenerative diseases of joints, such as osteoarthritis, by slowing destruction and damage to cartilage and joints; decreasing inflammation and preventing inflammatory-induced destructive processes from occurring; and possibly affecting levels of pain stimulators..

Gamma-linolenic Acid (GLA) Reduces Inflammation and Stiffness

Dr. Marya Zilberberg, in her review of close to 40 clinical papers on GLA, notes that GLA consistently reduces inflammation and joint stiffness without any of the serious side effects associated with pharmaceutical drugs. "We saw about a 60 to 65 percent reduction in morning stiffness for these patients," said Zilberg. "In other words if you have two hours of morning stiffness, there is a 1.5 hour reduction compared to a 6.7 minute reduction with a fake pill. It is an extremely striking difference."

This is good news for those with arthritis and inflammatory disorders who see morning stiffness as the most debilitating effect of their disease. "If you were to ask an arthritis patient about morning stiffness, you would find that it is an extremely important indicator of how their disease is doing," said Zilberberg. These results demonstrate the importance of long-term supplementation with large doses of GLA from borage or evening primrose oil for osteoarthritis and rheumatoid arthritis.

GLA Reduces the Use of NSAIDs: Recent research suggests that use of GLA reduces the immune factors that promote inflammation and joint tissue injuries. It is important to decrease these dangerous immune factors in order to reduce cartilage damage (the event that leads to bone erosion and crippling) and joint swelling in patients suffering from rheumatoid arthritis (RA).

Supplementing with GLA not only decreases the clinical symptoms of RA, but taking GLA can reduce the side effects of NSAIDs by repairing damage to the stomach lining. Studies show that GLA protects the stomach lining from the gastric acid that could cause stomach ulcers due to repeated or overuse of NSAIDs. As early as 1988, researchers confirmed that daily supplementation with 540 mg of GLA from evening primrose oil could help patients reduce their use of NSAIDs and therefore protect their stomach linings. At the beginning of the study, 100 percent of patients were on their full NSAID dosage; after three months of supplementing with evening primrose oil, 70 percent of patients were still taking NSAIDs, and after six months, only 30 percent of patients were still taking NSAID at full dosage. This is a remarkable 70 percent reduction in patients using NSAIDs.

GLAs and Rheumatoid Arthritis: The Omega-6 fatty acid GLA found in evening primrose oil and borage oil is useful in the management of rheumatoid arthritis; it reduces pain and inflammation. Arachidonic acid (found primarily in organ and red meat, eggs and dairy products) produces inflammatory compounds. Supplementing with GLA-rich evening primrose oil or borage oil helps to reduce the inflammatory by-products from arachidonic acid. GLA helps to suppress the inflammatory immune cells and the synovial cell proliferation in inflamed synovial tissue; this will help decrease inflammation and pain. In clinical trials, GLA has been shown to replace pharmaceutical drugs as an NSAID substitute and, in fact, might function as a disease-modifying anti-rheumatic drug.

GLA for Juvenile Rheumatoid Arthritis: Data from a recent study conducted at the Shriners Hospital for Children in Springfield, Massachusetts found that borage oil can benefit children with Juvenile Rheumatoid Arthritis (JRA). Preliminary data from the study was presented by lead researcher Deborah Rothman, MD, PhD, during the Annual Meeting of the American College of Rheumatology in Boston. In her research, Dr. Rothman found that the effects of borage oil were strongest for patients with polyarthritis.

The use of borage oil in cases of JRA may allow some patients to reduce their dosage of standard medications such as NSAIDs or corticosteroids. Children with rheumatic disease receiving long-term corticosteroids are at high risk of developing osteoporosis and infections. Reduction of symptoms may be observed after one month of supplementation. The full effects of GLA supplementation are seen over longer periods.

Fish Oils (Omega-3 EPA and DHA)
The first scientific paper describing the use of fish oil for treating

rheumatoid arthritis was published in the 18th century. Since then, laboratory and clinical studies have revealed the beneficial effects of fish oil on various forms of arthritis. The benefits were attributed to the Omega-3 fatty acids EPA and DHA. EPA and DHA are incorporated into the cellular membranes and compete with arachidonic acid for the enzymes responsible for the production of anti-inflammatory prostaglandins.

Eicosapentaenoic acid (EPA) and Docosahexaenoic Acid (DHA) are found in high amounts in cold-water fish. EPA and DHA can also be converted from flaxseed oil, albeit in poor amounts. It is estimated that the conversion rate of flaxseed oil to EPA and DHA is somewhere around 11 percent, meaning you would have to consume a lot of flaxseed oil to get the equivalent amount of DHA and EPA found in fish oils. DHA and EPA have powerful anti-inflammatory properties. Eat at least 3 to 5 servings of salmon, herring, mackerel or tuna per week. If you are unable to eat fish or dislike the taste, use pharmaceutical grade fish oil capsules from wild salmon or small fish including sardine, mackerel or herring. Michael Murray, N.D. was one of the experts who coined the term "pharmaceutical grade fish oil." In order for fish oil to be pharmaceutical grade, it must possess the following characteristics:

- It must be manufactured in a certified GMP-facility (Good Manufacturing Practices, which are governed by strict regulatory rules) approved for pharmaceutical products.
- It must be manufactured according to pharmaceutical standards that include quality control steps to ensure the product is free from lipid peroxides, heavy metals, environmental contaminants and other harmful compounds.
- It must provide at least a 60 percent concentration of the most active long-chain Omega-3 fatty acids (EPA and DHA).
- The ratio of Omega-3 fatty acids to arachidonic acid must be greater than 50:1.

- It must contain the optimal amount of natural vitamin E as a preservative.
- Studies show that Omega-3s decrease inflammation and degradation and help to prevent the cartilage damage that occurs in the joints. This can slow the progression of degenerative joint diseases, such as osteoarthritis.

EPA and DHA reduce the formation of bad prostaglandins and regulate immune factor production, which controls how long, how fast and how much the immune system acts or reacts. EPA produces the anti-inflammatory prostaglandins (good guys). Fish oils improve joint mobility and reduce the severity of pain and inflammation without any short- or long-term side-effects.

Abnormalities of fatty acid composition in synovial fluid in the joints have been documented in rheumatoid arthritis patients. In a 1999 study of 39 arthritic patients, synovial cell fluid samples were obtained from nine of the patients. Decreased levels of EPA and total Omega-3 fatty acids were observed in the blood and joint fluid of patients with rheumatoid arthritis. The researchers concluded that the fatty acid pattern found in those who suffer from rheumatoid arthritis (decreased levels of Omega-3s) may explain the beneficial effect of fish oil.

A 1998 review of the research confirmed the beneficial effects of fish oil in the treatment of arthritis. Fish oil reduces arthritis symptoms such as pain, number of affected joints and morning stiffness in a dose-dependent manner. Clinical benefits were seen after twelve weeks, with a dosage of 3 g of EPA and DHA per day.

It also appears that fish oil will help arthritis sufferers reduce the amount of NSAIDs needed, and some patients may be able to discontinue use completely. The first study of fish oil and RA patients examined NSAID requirements in 37 of 64 patients who were given fish oil at a dose of 1.7 g per day of EPA and 1.1 g per day of DHA in a randomized, double-blind study. After six weeks of therapy, patients were advised to reduce their NSAID dose slowly. At 12 months, all fish-oil-treated patients were crossed over to a fake pill and assessed again three months later. At the three-month mark, a 41 percent reduction in NSAID usage was achieved. Overall, patients taking fish oil had a dramatic reduction in their symptoms.

Combining EPA and GLA

Some research has studied the use of EPA and GLA together and their impact on reducing pro-inflammatory substances. A study at Wake Forest University School of Medicine found that patients supplementing with a combination of EPA and GLA reduced production of pro-inflammatory substances. A research review in *Lipids*, conducted at the University of Southampton, England noted that taking EPA and GLA supplements decreased the production of the pro-inflammatory immune factors that cause swelling, pain, redness and heat in the joints.

GLUCOSAMINE SULPHATE

Touted as the "Arthritis Cure," glucosamine (pronounced glue-*cose*-a-mean) sulphate has been shown, in more than a dozen human trials, to be as good as or better than non-steroidal anti-inflammatory drugs (NSAIDs) in controlling pain and inflammation. Glucosamine normalizes cartilage metabolism while stopping its breakdown and acts as a shock absorber by lubricating and repairing joint tissue. It is an important constituent of bone and cartilage, skin, hair and nails. Several studies have shown that doses of glucosamine sulphate reduce the pain and inflammation caused by arthritis-induced joint destruction. Researchers around the world have compared the effectiveness of glucosamine to the common pain reliever ibuprofen (Advil®, Motrin® and Nuprin, etc.). Double-blind, placebo-controlled studies verified that glucosamine was dramatically better at controlling both pain and inflammation than ibuprofen. Pain and inflammation were reduced even after the glucosamine was no longer consumed. In addition, glucosamine has the amazing ability to aid the rebuilding process of the cartilage matrix that makes up our joint tissue.

Celadrin and Glucosamine Combined

Use Celadrin to stop the inflammatory process that is causing joint destruction and add glucosamine sulphate to repair the damage that has already occurred. Celadrin is effective at halting the joint-damaging process (whether due to RA or OA), while glucosamine can repair damage already done to those joints affected. Celadrin works by providing continuous lubrication and allowing the cell membrane to repel inflammatory messengers from the immune system. It also stops the cascade of inflammation and the assaults on the membrane, which cause stiffness. Celadrin helps glucosamine perform faster and more efficiently in building joint cartilage. The dual action of Celadrin and glucosamine will provide rapid joint cushioning, quickly alleviate inflammation, build cartilage and restore the entire joint area. Cartilage repair usually begins within two months. Spectacular results have been experienced by those individuals with RA who have adopted the combination treatment.

GREEN-LIPPED MUSSEL EXTRACT

Green-lipped mussel (*Perna canaliculus*) is a New Zealand shellfish; an extract from this mollusk has been shown to inhibit inflammation in cases of rheumatoid arthritis and osteoarthritis. Not all research using green-lipped mussel for OA and RA has demonstrated therapeutic benefits, but some has been positive.

In one trial, both freeze-dried powder and lipid extract of green-lipped mussel were effective at reducing symptoms in 70 percent of people with OA and 76 percent of people with RA. A similar study of people with either OA or RA showed green-lipped mussel extract reduced pain in 50 percent and 67 percent of the patients respectively, after three months of supplementation. In 1986, stabilized dried mussel extracts became available.

Earlier studies had found no beneficial effect of green-lipped mussel extract on arthritis, but all used preparations that had not been stabilized, a fact that may help explain some of the discrepancies in the research. One recent animal study compared the two forms and found a stabilized lipid extract to be significantly more effective than a non-stabilized extract at inhibiting inflammation. Because both forms are currently available on the market, check the label to see which one you are using.

One animal study found that green-lipped mussel extract also significantly reduced stomach ulcers resulting from taking NSAIDs. In a double-blind study of people with asthma, supplementation with a proprietary extract of New Zealand green-lipped mussel (Lyprinol) twice a day for eight weeks significantly decreased daytime wheezing and improved airflow through the bronchi. *Those with shellfish allergies should avoid this product. Nausea was noted in some taking high doses.*

MSM (METHYL-SULFONYL-METHANE)
According to the authors of MSM, *The Natural Solution for Pain*, MSM relieves pain, reduces inflammation and IL-1, reduces scar tissue formation, reduces muscle spasms and more. MSM is a major source of sulfur in humans. Sulfur is especially important for healthy joint function. It stabilizes the connective tissue matrix of cartilage, tendons and ligaments. As early as the

1930s, researchers found that arthritic patients were deficient in this essential nutrient. By simply adding sulfur to the diet, arthritis symptoms improved. Sulfur also promotes proper liver function and improves insulin's action.

Michael Murray, N.D. states that, "MSM provides significant advantages over other forms of sulfur in that it is completely safe. When people say they are allergic to sulfur, what they really mean is that they are allergic to the so-called sulfa drugs or sulfite-containing food additives. It is impossible to be allergic to sulfur as sulfur is an essential mineral."

Research reported in *The Journal of Anti-aging Medicine* found that when eight patients were given 2,250 mg of MSM daily and six patients were given a placebo, after six weeks of treatment those taking MSM indicated they had better than 80 percent reduction in pain.

PEPTACE™
Although it is not an anti-inflammatory, PeptAce is the most effective natural substance for lowering blood pressure and is recommended in the Heart Disease section. PeptAce is a mixture of 9 small peptides (proteins) derived from bonito (a member of the tuna family). It works to lower blood pressure by inhibiting ACE (angiotensin converting enzyme), thereby inhibiting the formation of angiotensin II, a substance that increases both the fluid volume and the degree of constriction of the blood vessels. If we use a garden hose model, angiotensin II would be similar to pinching off the hose while turning up the faucet full blast. By inhibiting the formation of this compound, anti-ACE peptides relax the arterial walls and reduce fluid volume. PeptAce fish peptides exert the strongest inhibition of ACE reported for any naturally occurring substance available.

Three major clinical studies have been conducted with PeptAce fish peptides. The material appears to be effective in about two-thirds of people with high blood pressure — about the same percentage that many prescription drugs achieve. The degree of blood pressure reduction in these studies was quite significant, typically reducing the systolic by at least 10 mm Hg and the diastolic by 7 mm Hg in people with borderline and mild hypertension. The typical dosage is three 500-mg capsules daily. No side effects were reported in the clinical studies, and a safety study showed no side effects with dosages as high as 30 g daily.

PeptAce fish peptides do not affect blood pressure in people without hypertension, do not interact negatively with potassium and have no adverse drug interactions, so they can be used in combination with conventional anti-hypertensive drugs.

TURMERIC (CURCUMIN)
Esteemed by Ayurvedic practitioners for centuries, turmeric contains anti-inflammatory curcuminoids. These reduce pain by blocking the enzymes that cause inflammation. Turmeric inhibits the breakdown of arachidonic acid. Several double-blind studies have shown dramatic improvements in symptoms experienced by rheumatoid arthritis sufferers. Turmeric is also an antioxidant. Researchers at the University of California found that curcumin, in both low and high doses, reduced the inflammatory immune factors IL-1 and IL-6 secreted by microglia cells. This finding means turmeric shows great promise for the prevention of Alzheimer's and memory decline.

VITAMINS
A study published in the June 26, 2002 *Journal of the American Medical Association* suggested that vitamins E, C, beta-carotene and a general multi-vitamin with minerals may help protect

people against cognitive and memory decline. Vitamins E and C are powerful anti-inflammatory nutrients inhibiting IL-1 and IL-6, so it makes sense that they would protect our brains from injury or inflammatory assault.

Vitamin A helps to increase the good immune factors that turn off the inflammatory and pain-causing immune factor IL-1. Vitamin D, the only vitamin that acts like a hormone, reduces IL-1 and -12. Vitamin E decreases inflammatory prostaglandins that are associated with pain and inflammation. It also decreases the negative effects of stress. (Stressors cause the release of our stress hormone, cortisol. Cortisol then causes the inflammatory immune factor IL-6 to be released.) Vitamin E also increases the good immune factors that keep IL-1 and IL-6 under control.

WATER
Yes, water cushions your joints. If you are not drinking six to ten glasses of water every day, your joint cushions are dehydrated. Water helps to eliminate all of the debris left over from inflammatory reactions as well, particularly in those with asthma and allergies.

WHITE WILLOW BARK
White willow bark is nature's aspirin. It is an ancient remedy used to treat fevers and arthritic complaints. Salicin is its active ingredient. Many human studies have evaluated White willow bark's ability to rapidly relieve pain and reduce inflammation.

One Final Note: Gentle Exercise for Weight Control

Our knees and hips bear up to ten times our body weight. Simply by managing your weight and losing as little as ten pounds, you can help reduce the pressure your weight-bearing joints must carry. Eat plenty of vegetables (omitting the foods that are associated with increasing inflammation); eliminate all sugar (do not use aspartame or sucrolose; instead use stevia or xylitol, both natural sweeteners that do not produce inflammation).

Gentle exercise is where you should begin, nothing too strenuous. Here are some tips to keep your muscles and joints healthy:

- Walk every day, even if only to the end of your driveway and back. Walk ten feet if that is all you can do.
- Join a beginner water fitness class. They are classed as "no impact" because the water provides you with a cushion. After your water fitness class, sit in the sauna and you will benefit from some detoxification through your skin, and your joints will enjoy the warmth.
- If you are able, do some weight-bearing exercises. Use light weights; half or one pound weights will do. Velcro weights that you wear strapped around your legs or arms are a great way to start weight-bearing exercise. An effective way to begin is to sit in a chair and flex your knee to slowly lift your legs up and down, and then slowly lift your arms up and down, from the shoulder. Do whatever works to get a little movement into your daily routine. Start with a few repetitions, and slowly build up to three sets of up to ten repetitions.
- Rest and do not become fatigued.
- Find some activity you love to do, such as gardening, walking or dancing.

Common Inflammatory Conditions

The following section provides an overview of some of the more common inflammatory conditions. Each condition is divided into sections, including an overview of the condition, symptoms, causes, a "Prescription for Health" that details natural treatments, plus health and lifestyle tips to enhance recovery. The supplements recommended are in order of importance. It is not necessary to take every nutrient suggested, but combinations of certain nutrients are very effective, for example Celadrin and glucosamine for arthritis. Many of the nutrient recommendations are for vitamins and minerals that you will find in your multivitamin with mineral supplement, so you won't be taking more than a few pills or capsules at a time. The more health tips and recommendations that you adopt, the faster you will progress on the road to optimal health.

Allergies

For most individuals, allergies are a seasonal or situational problem causing unbearable symptoms. The pollens of spring or a friend's cat may be the reason for itchy eyes, runny nose, sneezing, wheezing and more. Yet for some people, allergy symptoms never seem to abate. They are a constant problem. Common environmental exposures and foods trigger allergies and promote asthmatic attacks. But why is it that only some are affected by allergies and others are not?

There are two types of allergic response: the first is the classic allergic response whereby the allergen (e.g., peanuts, pollen, shellfish or pet dander) triggers an increase in immunoglobulin E (IgE). The reaction is immediate and easily determined by a blood test that will show a high count of IgE antibodies. The IgE antibodies meet an invader and trigger the release of inflammatory messengers (including histamine) from mast cells to kill or immobilize the invader. Allergies that are characterised by IgE antibodies are called atopic. Allergens can initiate different symptoms depending on which area of the body they settle in. An upper respiratory tract irritation will feature sneezing and a runny nose, while the same allergen in the lower respiratory tract will produce wheezing or coughing.

The second type of allergic response is a cell-mediated or delayed-onset response. They are more difficult to diagnose because the symptoms may not occur immediately. An increase in IgG antibodies is associated with delayed-onset allergies. The symptoms tend to originate in the gastrointestinal tract and be in the form of gastric upsets, diarrhea, irritable bowel, hyperactivity (in children) and brain fog-type symptoms.

Many illnesses, including autoimmune disorders, arthritis and other inflammatory diseases and attention deficit hyperactivity disorder are associated with or arise from years of untreated or hidden allergies.

SYMPTOMS

Allergies can elicit a cornucopia of symptoms that are so wide and varied that it can be difficult to detect an allergy over some other condition. Common reactions are sneezing, watery eyes, runny nose, itching, dermatitis, earache, congested nasal passages, headaches, hives, bloating, blurred vision, cramps, frequent urination, stomach distress, diarrhea, gas, edema, fatigue, depression, brain fog, lack of concentration, poor memory, anxiety, feeling faint, hyperactivity, insomnia, irritability, arthritic pain or muscle pain. Other symptoms include dark circles under the eyes, red or burning ears, constant nose rubbing (some allergic people have a crease just above the bulb of their nose from chronic rubbing or one nostril will be stretched in the direction of the rub), inflamed tonsils and recurrent throat infections, skin rashes, eczema, constipation, nausea, bloated stomach, heartburn, excessive sweating, extreme salivation, bedwetting in children or mood swings.

CAUSES

The immune system is causing the allergic symptoms in its bid to rid the body of what it sees as invaders. This is not a normal response and occurs only in those individuals who have a hyper-stimulated or overly sensitive immune system. In an allergy-prone person, when the immune system encounters an allergen such as pollen, a certain cell called the T-helper-2 cell releases an immune factor called Interleukin-4 (IL-4). Interleukin-4 causes B cells to secrete IgE antibodies that then attach to mast cells. Mast cells release a cascade of chemicals (including histamine) that promotes allergic symptoms. Gamma interferon is also reduced in allergic persons; gamma interferon is responsible for stopping IL-4. Without adequate interferon, the allergic reaction is not controlled. Histamine is responsible for the symptoms like watery eyes, itchy skin and more. In asthmatics, the situation is even worse because not only does the immune system release Interleukin-4, but also an immune factor called Interleukin-6 (IL-6). Interleukin-6 in asthmatics causes lung tissue damage and, if not controlled, can lead to reliance on steroid medications and puffers. The key to halting allergies in their tracks is stopping the release of Interleukin-4 and controlling Interleukin-6.

PRESCRIPTION FOR HEALTH

Nutrient	Dosage	Action
Multivitamin with minerals, including: Vitamin B6 in the form P5P: 60 mg per day Vitamin B12 (methylcobalamin): 1000 mcg Vitamin C: 1000 mg	As directed	Provides nutrient foundation; repairs mucous membranes damaged by allergy; reduces severity and occurrence of allergy attacks
Celadrin™	1500 mg tablet/capsule form or 1050 mg soft gel, per day	Inhibits immune factors that promote the allergic response
Quercetin	500-1000 mg, two to three times per day (Children five to 12 years of age: half the dosage)	Stops histamine release; anti-allergenic; antioxidant; especially effective for those sensitive to airborne allergens
Fish oil (pharmaceutical grade)	3000 mg per day	Inhibits inflammation
Magnesium	500 mg, three times per day	Acts as a bronchodilator and antihistamine; reduces stress
Aller-7™	660 mg, twice per day, with meals for 12 weeks; then 330 mg per day thereafter	Promotes a healthy immune system and respiratory tract; stabilizes mast cells to control inflammation; neutralizes free radicals
Enzymes (Zymactive™)	1-2 capsules with each meal	Aids digestion; helps minimize food allergies; helps to repair leaky gut
BB536 Bifidobacterium longum	1-2 capsules per day	Improves intestinal flora; helps those with food allergies and asthma
Pantethine	300 mg, twice per day	Reduces sensitivity to aldehydes

HEALTH TIPS TO ENHANCE HEALING

- Avoid allergens whenever possible.
- Start a diet diary and write down everything you eat to see if there is any correlation to your allergy symptoms. Ask for a referral to an allergy specialist and get tested for possible triggers. Some allergies may only be detected with the help of an ELISA (Enzyme-Linked Immunosorbent Assay) test.
- Avoid sulfite-containing foods. Beer and wine commonly contain sulfites.
- Drink at least 8 to 10 glasses of pure, clean, filtered water each day because water controls histamine production. For every juice or caffeine beverage you drink, add another glass of water.
- Rotate the foods you eat; never eat the same foods every day. Consume a diet that emphasizes natural, whole foods such as legumes, fresh fruit and vegetables, fish, healthy fats and oils and nuts and seeds.
- Avoid processed or junk foods because they contain chemicals that stress the body and have no nutritional value.
- Use cayenne, onions and garlic as much as possible as they are high in quercetin.
- Stress can aggravate allergies, so get plenty of rest and relaxation.

OTHER RECOMMENDATIONS

- If you smoke, stop now. If you don't smoke, but are exposed to secondhand smoke, remove yourself from the situation or ask people to butt out. Secondhand smoke has 4,000 chemicals in it, including known carcinogens. Smoke that wafts from the lit end does not go through a filter and is more poisonous than what is inhaled by the smoker. Children raised in environments where there is smoking are more prone to allergies and asthma.
- If attacks are brought on by airborne allergens, make your living environment as allergen-free as possible. Wash all

bedding and blankets weekly; get rid of carpets; vacuum and dust with a damp cloth often; do not allow pets up on the furniture. Furniture should have washable slipcovers. You may also want to have your home checked for environmental hazards such as lead and asbestos.

■ When using herbal remedies, keep in mind that the herbs may belong to the same plant family as your allergens. For example, if you have an allergy to legumes, you may have a reaction to red clover, soybean extracts or astragalus.

■ Men with mustaches may be aggravating their airborne allergies because allergens build up on the surface of the mustache.

Also see *Asthma*

Arthritis

Millions of people suffer from one form of arthritis or another and, contrary to popular belief, it is not a disease affecting only the elderly. Some forms of arthritis strike toddlers, while thousands of others are stricken in the prime of their lives. Arthritis is the most prevalent chronic condition affecting women, particularly between the ages of 20 and 40. The U.S. National Institute of Arthritis and Musculoskeletal and Skin Diseases reports that one in seven Americans has some form of arthritis.

Arthritis ("arth" meaning joint; "itis" meaning inflammation) consists of over 100 different conditions, from gout to rheumatoid arthritis (see box below for a partial list). Although most of these disorders involve joint or muscle inflammation, others, like lupus, involve the skin, lungs and kidney. Inflammation, swelling and, most importantly, pain are hallmarks of arthritis.

Osteoarthritis, the most common form of arthritis, is a gradual wearing away of the cartilage that cushions the joints by preventing the bones from scraping against each other. New research is also finding that osteoarthritis occurs when the ability to regenerate normal cartilage is impaired. Repetitive activities and sports injuries, as well as aging, are associated with the development of osteoarthritis.

Rheumatoid arthritis (RA), the second most common form, is an autoimmune disease. The immune system produces antibodies that destroy the synovium membranes around the lubricating fluid in the joints. RA may begin in fits and starts, taking months or years to progress, but for about 25 percent of sufferers, it begins abruptly and is severe. Correcting imbalances in the immune system is the focus of treatment.

TYPES OF ARTHRITIS

- Ankylosing Spondylitis
- Gout (see *Gout*)
- Infective Arthritis
- Juvenile Chronic Arthritis
- Osteoarthritis (the most common type)
- Polymyalgia Rheumatica
- Pseudo Gout (see *Gout*)
- Psoriatic Arthritis (see *Psoriasis*)
- Raynaud's Phenomenon (see *Raynaud's Disease/Phenomenon*)
- Reiter's Disease
- Rheumatoid Arthritis
- Sjogren's Syndrome (see *Sjogren's Syndrome*)
- Systemic Lupus Erythematosus (see *Systemic Lupus Erythematosus*)

SYMPTOMS

Osteoarthritis: Usually osteoarthritis appears after the age of forty and is characterized by joint pain and stiffness that increases in severity over a long period of time. Scientists now believe that this form of arthritis may actually begin as early as age 20 or 30 and that we only notice the symptoms in our 40s and beyond. The joints may become swollen and lose their mobility. After much of the cartilage has been worn away, bone spurs develop in the joint spaces.

Rheumatoid Arthritis: The joint pain and stiffness of RA is more noticeable in the morning and, like osteoarthritis, the joints become swollen. Unlike osteoarthritis, however, RA can strike suddenly and at any time of life, even in childhood (Juvenile Rheumatoid Arthritis). Other symptoms include fatigue, fever, depression, anemia, weight loss and night sweats. When the joints are inflamed, they take on a purplish color and, as the disease progresses, the hands and feet become deformed. RA attacks symmetrically, afflicting both wrists, ankles or both knees. In order to confirm a diagnosis of RA, four out of the following seven criteria must be met: morning stiffness that lasts more than an hour; the arthritis is symmetrical; three joint areas simultaneously inflamed (not just bony overgrowth); arthritis is present in any of the hand joints; nodules lay under the skin on bony prominences; serum rheumatoid factor levels are abnormal; and erosions or decalcification are detected by X-ray.

CAUSES

Osteoarthritis: Better known as "wear and tear" arthritis, as the nickname suggests, it can arise from repetitive use or abuse of the joints from heavy labor, sports and injuries. Obesity aggravates arthritis because greater strain is put on the joints. Poor nutrition and dehydration as well as certain foods and environmental allergies can contribute to the condition. Aging is usually cited as a factor (70 percent of the elderly have it), and there is an assumption that it is an inevitable aspect of aging. This is not true. If care is taken to address the other factors, then you may live a long life without osteoarthritis.

Doctors used to think that arthritis was all about damaged or defective cartilage. Now they understand that cartilage is important but tendons, muscles, ligaments and bones also play a role in the development of osteoarthritis. We also now know that some cartilage is more resistant to damage; our ankles, for example, rarely develop osteoarthritis. The wrist develops arthritis less often than the base joint of the thumb. Women with strong, healthy bones (free of osteoporosis) are at a greater risk of developing osteoarthritis. Scientist suspect that the bio-chemical process that helps increase the repair rate in bone causes damage to cartilage.

Or could it be that weakened muscles contribute to osteoarthritis? Research by Dr. Kenneth Brandt, a rheumatologist at Indiana University in Indianapolis, studied a group of 400 elderly patients. He found that weakness in the quadriceps (the large muscle on the front of the thighs that helps raise and lower the leg) in most cases preceded the development of osteoarthritis. He also found that the stronger the muscle, the less the load of body weight that was bearing on the joint; this factor reduced damage to cartilage. Walking and other weight-bearing exercise may be an even more important preventative factor than was previously thought.

Once osteoarthritis has begun, the immune system becomes the engine of joint damage by sending out immune messengers that destroy cartilage and bone.

Rheumatoid Arthritis (RA): Stress and its ability to affect the hormones that promote inflammation, allergies, heredity, obesity, nutritional deficiencies, some vaccines, a hyperactive immune system and even viral or bacterial infections are just a few of the potential causes of RA. Ten years ago rheumatologists would have disagreed that these factors play a role in promoting arthritis, but new research has shown otherwise.

PRESCRIPTION FOR HEALTH
There are many nutrients that have been clinically proven to aid the treatment of arthritis. I have listed the different options in order of importance; first try Celadrin and add glucosamine, if you wish.

Nutrient	Dosage	Action
Multivitamin and mineral supplement containing a minimum of: vitamin A: 5000 IU vitamin D: 400 IU vitamin C: 1000 mg vitamin E: 200 IU B complex vitamin B12: (methylcobalamin) 1000 mcg	Use as directed	Provides a solid nutrient foundation that supports muscle, cartilage and bone development; helps support healthy immune function; and controls inflammatory factors. Also aids the synthesis of collagen, the glue-like substance in cartilage, and reduces pain.
Celadrin™	Orally: 1500 mg tablet/ capsule form or 1050 mg soft gel, per day Topical cream: apply twice each day	Reduces swelling and pain; improves joint mobility; inhibits inflammation and joint destruction
Glucosamine sulphate	500 mg, three times per day	Repairs cartilage; combine with Celadrin
Fish oil (pharmaceutical grade)	3000 mg per day	Reduces hormones (eicosanoids) responsible for increasing inflammation; prevents cartilage damage; reduces associated pain

Nutrient	Dosage	Action
GLA from evening primrose oil or borage oil	Adults: 2000 mg of borage or 4000 mg of evening primrose oil per day Children: 500-1000 mg of borage oil or 1000-2000 mg of evening primrose oil per day	Relieves pain, inflammation and morning joint stiffness. (Studies show reduced need for NSAIDs.)
Turmeric (curcumin)	200 mg, three times per day	Anti-inflammatory
Enzymes (Zymactive™) (proteolytic enzmes)	3 capsules per day, between meals, on an empty stomach	Reduces inflammation in the joints; controls immune functions that further destroy joint tissue
SAM-e S-adenosyl-methionine (sulfur compound)	200 mg, twice per day	Reduces pain and inflammation; promotes proteoglycan production
DHEA	Have your doctor do a DHEAs test to see if you are deficient. If so, take 5-10 mg per day *(Not recommended for those at risk of estrogen-receptor positive cancers)*	Reduces IL-6; normalizes cortisol; stops inflammatory processes
Boswellia	Standardized dose of 200-400 mg, three times per day	Anti-inflammatory; as effective as NSAIDs
MSM	1-2 grams per day	Anti-inflammatory
Devil's claw	1-2 grams per day	Anti-inflammatory
Bromelain (contains sulfur and proteolytic enzymes)	2000-6000 mcu (1300-4000 gdu) per day, on an empty stomach	Anti-inflammatory; improves joint mobility; reduces swelling
White willow bark (standardized)	As directed	Reduces pain and inflammation

HEALTH TIPS TO ENHANCE HEALING

- Drink 8 to 10 glasses of pure, clean, filtered water every day to keep your joint cushions from becoming dehydrated. For every juice or caffeine beverage that you consume, you must have another glass of water.
- Avoid these foods to prevent flare-ups: citrus fruit, milk, organ meats, red meat, sugar products, salt, paprika and cayenne pepper, tobacco and any member of the nightshade family (potatoes, eggplant, tomatoes, peppers, etc.).
- Focus your diet on natural, whole foods: fresh fruit, vegetables, legumes, whole grains, healthy fats and oils, seafood and fresh fish. They are key to halting inflammation at the source. Eat foods rich in sulfur, including garlic, onions and asparagus.
- Non-weight-bearing exercise like water aerobics, swimming, stationary cycling and yoga should be performed. Be careful not to overburden joints or cause further pain and inflammation.
- If you are overweight, lose the excess. Even 10 extra pounds can put an additional 40 pounds of pressure on your arthritic knee and ankle joints.

OTHER RECOMMENDATIONS

- Use hot or cold compresses on the area to alleviate pain and inflammation.
- Take hot baths or saunas to keep the joints warm.
- Use topical ointments including Celadrin, capsaicin, menthol, dimethyl sulfoxide (DMSO) or quaternary amines. Look for capsaicin creams containing 0.025 to 0.075 percent capsaicin or menthol; both are soothing to sore joints (avoid contact with eyes).
- Start a diet diary; write down everything that you eat to see if there is any correlation with your arthritis symptoms. Ask for a referral to an allergy specialist and get tested for possible triggers. Some allergies may only be detected with the help of

an ELISA (Enzyme-Linked Immunosorbent Assay) test. Once you know what you are allergic to, avoid those allergens.

■ Beware of taking nonsteroidal anti-inflammatory drugs (NSAIDs), Celebrex, aspirin or acetaminophen long term; all of them promote digestive problems. See *Conventional Treatments*, page 12.

■ If you are taking methotrexate, you must supplement with B vitamins and folic acid as the drug reduces these nutrients, promoting nausea and diarrhea. Pernicious anemia may develop if the deficiency is not addressed

Pets and Arthritis

As the owner of two beautiful Bengal cats, one with osteoarthritis caused by hip dysplasia, I know how I feel when one of them is sick or in pain. Osteoarthritis in domestic animals is a common condition. Over 20 percent of dogs over the age of one are suffering this painful, debilitating condition. The causes of arthritis in pets are very similar to those in humans: poor nutrition, repetitive wear and tear on the joints and hereditary conditions associated with joint destruction. The family pet has also become the latest victim of inactivity and obesity. Overweight animals suffer more bouts of osteoarthritis.

Veterinarians use aspirin or acetaminophen or NSAID medications. The most common side effect of NSAID administration in dogs is gastrointestinal toxicity ranging from vomiting and diarrhea to a silent ulcer. Pet owners are leery of these drugs due to their side effects and they should be. There are far more contraindications for these drugs for animals than there are for humans. This has caused a shift to alternative therapies for the treatment of osteoarthritis in animals. The most common treatment is glucosamine sulphate, yet there is limited information showing its efficacy in dogs. Research using Celadrin in humans, rats and dogs shows great improvement in the joints within a relatively short period of time.

In 2001, results of a clinical trial using Celadrin for osteoarthritis in dogs was presented at the prestigious Experimental Biology Conference. An independent veterinary clinic was enlisted to conduct the study. Before taking part in the study, dogs had a physical exam, and blood and urine samples were taken for analysis. Both small and large dogs were included in the study, regardless of the current arthritis medication. The dogs were assessed at the beginning of the study and again 30 days later. Daily each dog was given dog chews containing Celadrin. A standard dose of two chews per 20 pounds was established. Twenty-four dogs between the ages of 8 and 13 years took part. Seventy-five percent of the owners noted improvement in stair climbing and gait. In addition, the dogs seemed more energetic, happier and to have a better temperament. There were no changes in blood or urine analysis.

Asthma

According to the American Lung Association, an estimated 16 million Americans are affected by asthma, a chronic lung condition characterized by inflammation of the airways. Among chronic illnesses in children, asthma is the most common, affecting twice as many boys as girls. Asthma severity may range from mild to life threatening, and over 6,000 people in North America die annually from the disease.

SYMPTOMS

Asthma is characterized by increased respiratory distress of the bronchi; as a result, airways become narrow and inflamed. Attacks begin with an excessive production of mucous, coughing, difficulty breathing and wheezing. The narrowing of the airway makes it extremely difficult for air to move in and out of the lungs. Recurring asthma "attacks" promote an abnormal thickening and hardening of air passages. The immune system also responds by secreting Interleukin-6, a dangerous immune factor that eventually destroys the delicate tissues lining the airway. When not suffering an asthma attack, an asthmatic will generally seem healthy.

CAUSES

Allergic reactions to foods or environmental triggers are present in over 50 percent of asthmatics. Heredity, allergens, nutritional deficiencies and an increase in the use of antibiotics in infants all contribute to the development of asthma. Car exhaust, petrochemicals, cigarette smoke, animal dander, molds, dust mites, flower and tree pollens and rising levels of air pollution are at the top of the environmental list of asthma triggers. The most common food allergies for asthmatics are wheat, milk, eggs, tomatoes and the sulfites found in beer and wine.

Several studies have looked at airborne allergen exposure during infancy in relation to asthma. Children raised in areas of low altitude have significantly higher rates of asthma. Moreover, children born during the high pollen months have a higher incidence of asthma and allergic rhinitis compared to those born during non-pollen production months. If you have a history of allergy or asthma, choosing low pollen months for the birth of your baby may be an important factor in protecting your child from future allergies.

Dairy allergy in children can cause ear infections that are unsuccessfully treated with repeated antibiotic therapy. Antibiotics create gut problems that eventually lead to "leaky gut" syndrome whereby undigested food particles enter the bloodstream through damaged areas of the gut, causing allergic reactions. Antibiotics are also associated with *Candida albicans* yeast overgrowth, which further exacerbates allergic symptoms. It becomes a vicious cycle of allergy, leaky gut problems, ear infections, antibiotics and *Candida* overgrowth.

Babies born to parents with food allergies should be breastfed for as long as possible. If a family history of dairy or wheat allergy exists, breastfeeding moms should avoid eating the allergy-causing foods to ensure that the child does not react to the antigens in breast milk. Chronic ear infections in young children are a good indicator of dairy allergy. Eliminate all dairy products, test for other allergies and see if ear infection rates decline.

The Antibiotic-Asthma Connection
Three or more courses of antibiotics in the first year of life are associated with a four-fold increase in the risk of asthma. Researchers at the University of Antwerp, Belgium have found a link between the use of antibiotics in the first year of life and an increased risk of developing asthma and allergic disorders in children who have a family history of allergy. Immunologists think that the proper development of our immune system and protection from allergies may be related to early exposure to certain natural infections, like colds and flu. (See *Health Fact* below for further information.)

What "Triggers" Asthma?
Most asthmatics have an allergy to some offending agent. This allergy then acts as the "trigger" that starts the inflammatory, lung-damaging asthma process. It is easy to diagnose an allergy that presents itself quickly and clearly in the form of a runny nose and itchy eyes after exposure to a particular agent such as cats or peanuts. It is much more difficult to discover an allergy that has vague symptoms or takes hours to display its effects (called delayed-onset allergy). (See *Allergies* for more information.)

Exercise Induced-Asthma

Some asthma attacks are triggered by exercise. Excessive coughing during exercise is an early warning sign that you may have asthma. Exercise should not be eliminated entirely, but milder forms of exercise should be adopted. Walk only on pollen-reduced days, breathe through the nose instead of the mouth and take extra vitamin C before starting physical activity.

PRESCRIPTION FOR HEALTH

If you are currently taking medication (including inhalers), do not stop treatment. Once you have been taking the nutrients below and adopting the protective measures, your symptoms will appear less often and with less intensity, requiring less medication.

Nutrient	Dosage	Action
Celadrin™	1500 mg tablet/capsule form or 1050 mg soft gel, per day	Powerful anti-inflammatory; inhibits immune factors that promote inflammation
Aller-7™	660 mg, twice per day with meals for 12 weeks; then 330 mg per day thereafter	Promotes a healthy immune system and respiratory tract; stabilizes mast cells to control inflammation; neutralizes free radicals
Vitamin B6 (taken with B complex)	50 mg per day	Repairs mucous membranes damaged by allergies; reduces allergic reactions
Vitamin B12	1000 mcg sublingal, twice per day or a 1000 mcg injection with folic acid, weekly for four weeks	Reduces or stops wheezing
Vitamin C	1000 mg, twice per day	Reduces severity and occurrence of allergy attacks; protects against exercise-induced asthma

Lycopene	10-30 mg per day	Protects against exercise-induced asthma; antioxidant
Quercetin	Adults: 500-1000 mg, two to three times per day Children five to 12: half the dosage	Works as an antihistamine, anti-allergenic and antioxidant; especially effective for those sensitive to airborne allergens
Magnesium	500 mg, three times per day	Stops attacks; acts as a bronchodilator and antihistamine; also required to replace magnesium depleted during an attack
Fish oil (pharmaceutical grade)	3000 mg per day	Reduces inflammation
BB536 Bifidobacterium longum	As directed	Improves intestinal flora; reduces allergic reactions
Ginkgo biloba	Adults: 120-140 mg standardized extract per day Children five and up: 60 mg maximum	Reduces wheezing, coughing, shortness of breath and frequency of attacks

HEALTH TIPS TO ENHANCE HEALING

- Start a diet diary; write down everything that you eat to see if there is any correlation with your asthma symptoms. Ask for a referral to an allergy specialist and get tested for possible triggers. Some allergies may only be detected with the help of an ELISA (Enzyme-Linked Immunosorbent Assay) test. I recommend Serammune Physicians Lab at 1-800-553-5472 for the ELISA/ACT allergy test to rule out delayed-onset allergies. Once you know what you are allergic to, avoid those allergens.

- Drink 8 to 10 glasses of pure, clean, filtered water every day to control histamine production.
- Stop smoking. See *Allergies* for more information on second hand smoke and asthma in children.

OTHER RECOMMENDATIONS

- Stay fit and lose any extra pounds. Carrying extra weight, especially on the upper torso, can decrease lung capacity and make it more difficult to breathe.
- Ninety percent of asthmatics are "mouth breathers" (versus breathing through the nose), making it easier for pollution, organisms and cold air to get into the lungs. Those with asthma are also often poor at exhaling the air from their lungs completely. Practice taking deep breaths in through your nose and then slowly expelling all the air out through your mouth. Do this exercise five times and repeat several times throughout the day.
- In North America, double-glazed windows, central heating and energy-efficient homes result in an overabundance of dust mites and molds, which exacerbate allergic asthma. Fresh air is essential and an attempt to have an allergen-free home can help reduce asthma attacks. See *Allergies* for additional tips.
- When using herbal remedies, keep in mind that the herbs may belong to the same plant family as your allergens.
- The use of two inhalers per month creates a higher risk for a lethal asthma attack. Misuse of inhalers is a serious concern. As inhaler use increases, so must the dosage as the body becomes tolerant over time. Excessive reliance on inhalers also increases the risk for heart problems, including high blood pressure and stroke.

Early Exposure to Infection May Stop Asthma

Professor Paolo Matricardi, of Rome, stated in *The British Medical Journal* that stomach infections early in childhood may help people avoid respiratory allergies and asthma later in life. Researchers believe that food-borne bacterial infections in childhood may help the immune system build up a resistance to allergies.

Many scientists believe that environmental poisons and pollution are only partly responsible for the increase in asthma. Matricardi and his research team showed that 1,659 air force cadets who had stomach flu early in life and exposure to food-borne bacteria and the common stomach bacteria *helicobacter pylori* were less likely to suffer asthma and upper respiratory infections.

Our fear of bacteria and obsession with cleanliness has gone overboard. Matricardi stated that "we must improve hygiene to reduce the impact of infectious diseases, but at the same time, we must learn how to safely train our immune system, especially during infancy, in order to prevent allergy." We must realize that childhood illnesses are the training ground for our immune systems. In order for the immune system to develop properly, a few illnesses in early childhood may be a good thing.

Did you know? Between 1980 and 1994, the number of children aged 4 years and under who suffer from asthma rose 300 percent. In children aged 5 to 14, the rate doubled.

Bowel Disease

Over 1.1 million North Americans suffer from inflammatory bowel disease (IBD); Canada has one of the highest rates of IBD in the world.

IBD is a general term used for Crohn's and ulcerative colitis where inflammation of the bowel causes anemia, fever and weight loss. It occurs in men and women equally, and tends to strike between the ages of 16 and 40. Three thousand cases of Crohn's disease are diagnosed in North America every year. In people with IBD, the immune system is unable to down-regulate the inflammatory response. The inflammation injures the epithelium (the outer layer of tissue in the gut and elsewhere), resulting in gastric distress (among other symptoms) and damage to the tissues.

Colitis, also called ulcerative colitis, is an inflammation of the colon that causes a continuous need to eliminate (diarrhea). It can be mild to severe.

Irritable Bowel Syndrome (IBS)

Irritable bowel syndrome, also called spastic colon, is when the large intestine spasms and prevents the passage of waste (constipation) or moves it along too quickly (diarrhea). Women are twice as likely as men to have IBS. The American College of Gastroenterology says that over 50 million Americans are suffering with irritable bowel syndrome. The International Foundation for Bowel Dysfunction says that IBS is second only to the common cold as a cause of absenteeism from work. IBS is often confused with colitis or Crohn's disease, but IBS does not have the inflammation associated with IBD. Nor is it as serious – IBS is an annoying disorder, but it is not a disease requiring surgery or strong medication.

SYMPTOMS

Although each bowel disease is different, the symptoms are so similar that a proper diagnosis can be difficult. Adding to the problem are the facts that the symptoms are not unusual and we have all experienced them at some time. However, if you have a regular history of heartburn, nausea, diarrhea, gas, bloating, belching, abdominal cramps, constipation or bowel movements that are in ribbons or small balls, these problems should be addressed to prevent more serious damage. Consult your physician immediately if you have rectal bleeding, fever, sharp abdominal pain or intestinal obstruction.

CAUSES

The exacerbation of bowel diseases and disorders is inextricably linked to fried, greasy foods; a low-fiber diet; a diet with too much processed foods; or eating too much food. When we treat our stomachs like garborators by eating junk foods and not chewing our food properly, the small and large intestines suffer the consequences. Stress aggravates the situation. In IBS, the cause is unknown, but depression, stress and food allergies are the main triggers. IBD is promoted by the immune system. New evidence has found that the inflammatory factors secreted by the immune system (IL-1, IL-6 and IL-8) are associated with the damage to the intestinal wall and increased inflammation seen in bowel disease. At this time it appears that increased IL-6 is associated with Crohn's disease, while higher levels of IL-8 are more characteristic of colitis.

In the case of Crohn's disease, John Hermon-Taylor, a researcher at St. Georges Medical School near London claims that 55 percent of dairy herds in Western Europe and America are infected with a bacterium called *mycobacterium paratuberculosis* (MAP), which can survive the pasteurization process currently used to sterilize milk. (Water supplies can also become infected from the run-off from cow manure that seeps into the soil and contaminates well water.) The normal pasteurization process heats milk to 72 degrees Celsius for 15 seconds. In order to kill the MAP bacterium, milk would need to be heated for double the time or 30 seconds. Although no definitive study has proven paratuberculosis causes Crohn's, specialists believe that the scientific evidence supporting the role of an infectious agent is mounting, and that Crohn's treatments should focus on eliminating milk and treating bacteria.

PRESCRIPTION FOR HEALTH

Nutrient	Dosage	Action
Celadrin™	1500 mg tablet/capsule form or 1050 mg soft gel, per day	Powerful anti-inflammatory; inhibits immune factors that promote inflammation
Vitamin B12, sublingual	1000 mcg per week; absorption is impaired in those with bowel problems	Offsets deficiency caused by damage to the walls of the intestinal tract
Multivitamin with minerals	As directed	Provides a solid nutrient foundation
Folic acid	1–5 mg per day	Stops chronic diarrhea. Not to be taken in doses higher than 400 mcg by those with epilepsy.
Vitamin D3	400 IU per day	Reduces inflammatory immune factors; restores deficiencies that could lead to bone disease
Vitamin C with quercetin	1000 mg vitamin C per day; 500 mg quercetin per day	Controls inflammation
Calcium and magnesium	1000 mg calcium per day; 500 mg magnesium per day	Is anti-inflammatory; restores possible deficiencies; helps to prevent colon cancer

Digestive enzymes (Zymactive™)	1-2 capsules 15 minutes before meals	Aids proper digestion; reduces inflammation in the gut
Iron	10 mg per day	Use only if diagnosed with anemia
BB536 Bifidobacterium longum	As directed	Improves intestinal flora; reduces diarrhea, irritable bowel, diverticulosis and constipation
L-glutamine	1000 mg per day	Supports health of villi (the surfaces that facilitate absorption in the intestine)
Fish Oil (pharmaceutical grade)	3000 mg per day	Reduces inflammation; EPA is thought to suppress the leukotriene responsible for signaling inflammation in the gut lining
Evening primrose oil	500 mg, twice per day	Reduces inflammation by inhibiting immune factors
Peppermint oil (enteric-coated capsules)	3-6 capsules per day	Reduces cramps; relieves gas; increases bile (used predominantly for those with IBS)

HEALTH TIPS TO ENHANCE HEALING

- Eliminate food allergies.
- Aid digestion by taking digestive plant enzymes with every meal. If you experience gas and bloating, and bowel movements don't improve, you may not be producing enough stomach acid to break down your food properly. Hydrochloric acid supplements with meals may alleviate this condition.
- Don't dilute your stomach acid or enzymes by drinking too many fluids during your meal.
- Eat 7 to 10 half-cup servings of organic fruits and vegetables every day. Steam your vegetables and take digestive enzymes. Do not eat white pasta, white rice or white flour, and opt for natural whole foods instead.

- Eat one half cup of plain yogurt with active cultures every day unless you are lactose intolerant. Lactose intolerance is a common cause of bowel problems. Stop all dairy products for six weeks and see if your gut distress is relieved. Fermented soy or rice milk are great alternatives and they come in many flavors.

- Drink water – 8 to 10 glasses of pure, clean, filtered water a day, but do not drink during meals or else you will dilute your digestive enzymes. For every cup of beverage with caffeine that you drink, add another glass of water.

- To spark your digestive juices, add fresh-squeezed lemon juice to a cup of herbal tea fifteen minutes before your meal. Coffee aggravates the gut, so switch to herbal tea or try green tea. Green tea has a third of coffee's caffeine and is rich in antioxidants.

- Taken alone or in combination, effective herbs to soothe your tummy include ginger, peppermint and fennel. Try the bitter herbs such as dandelion, plantain, yarrow, wormwood or gentian or use Swedish Bitters before you eat.

- Big meals are hard to digest, so try eating small meals throughout the day. Not only will this help heal stomach problems, it will keep your blood sugar in a healthy range. Sit, relax and enjoy your food – remember that digestion begins in your mouth.

- Reduce stress. Do whatever it takes to reduce your stress levels. Meditation, yoga, breathing exercises and/or a walk in the park can help reduce the intestinal affects of stress.

- Using non-steroidal anti-inflammatory drugs (NSAIDs) can result in upper gastrointestinal ulcers, bleeding and digestive difficulties. There are many safe alternatives to NSAIDs. See *Natural Remedies* discussed at the front of this book.

- Avoid diet drinks because they usually contain aspartame, a substance containing known toxins. Sorbitol and other artificial sweeteners can create gas, bloating and increased diarrhea; white sugar depresses immunity. Try using the herbal sweeteners stevia or xylitol instead; they are available at the health food store.

■ Exercise regularly. Yoga or t'ai chi are great for improving circulation, reducing tension and promoting healthy digestion and elimination. Stretching exercises where you must touch your toes or draw your knees up to your chest are also good to get the bowels moving.

■ A chiropractor may be able to provide some relief, if there is a misalignment in your spine.

■ An acupuncturist may be able to provide relief and reduce the need for surgery.

Health Fact

Dr. Sherry Rogers, in her book *No More Heartburn* (Kensington Books, 2000), says 90 percent of gut problems can be alleviated with simple dietary changes, the elimination of allergy-causing foods and *Candida albicans*, stress reduction and immune enhancement.

Eczema (Atopic Dermatitis)

Eczema is an allergic condition whereby abnormalities in the immune system promote an overproduction of inflammatory and allergic reactions in the skin. This leads to poor resistance to skin bacteria and viruses. It is estimated that 10 percent of North Americans suffer from eczema. It is common in infants and toddlers and often appears when the child is teething or after immunizations. There are five types of eczema: Atopic (allergic), infantile seborrheic, adult seborrheic, occupational irritant contact and allergic contact dermatitis.

SYMPTOMS

Eczema is intensely itchy, and the skin may be flaky, thick, scaly, weeping or crusting, or it may change in color. The skin inflammation commonly appears on the wrists, ankles, face, and the creases of the knees, ears, between the fingers and on the elbows. Skin thickening often occurs after much scratching and rubbing, and bacterial or viral infections are also common.

CAUSES

Children are more likely to develop eczema if there is a history of asthma, eczema or hayfever in the family. Triggers include stress, infections and climate changes. Stress is a major factor in adult eczema flare-ups. Those with eczema often have allergies, proven by allergy tests and elevated IgE levels, as well as a family history of the condition. Common allergens are food additives and preservatives, milk, eggs, wheat, soy, tomatoes, oranges and peanuts. Eczema can be the result of other conditions such as *Candida albicans*, leaky gut syndrome and a lack of stomach acid. Those with eczema often have poor digestion, which increases allergic reactions. Severe essential fatty acid deficiency is also associated with the development of eczema, with the skin unable to hold moisture properly.

In occupational irritant contact and allergic contact dermatitis, exposure to environmental allergens such metal alloys in zippers and jewelry, cosmetics, perfumes, rubber, latex and poison ivy are the source of the problem. Infantile seborrhea is more commonly known as cradle cap and adult seborrhea is red, dry, flaky skin that may also appear as mild dandruff.

PRESCRIPTION FOR HEALTH

Nutrient	Dosage	Action
Celadrin™	Orally: 1500 mg tablet/ capsule form or 1050 mg soft gel, per day Topical cream: apply twice each day if skin is not broken	Powerful anti-inflammatory; inhibits immune factors that promote inflammation in the skin
Fish oil (pharmaceutical grade)	Adults: 3000 mg per day Children five to 12: use Learning Factors as directed	Controls inflammatory prostaglandins; ensures adequate EFA levels; maintains skin integrity
Multivitamin with minerals (for adults)	As directed	Provides a solid nutrient foundation
GLA from evening primrose oil or borage oil	Adults: 2000 mg of borage or 4000 mg of evening primrose oil per day Children: 500-1000 mg of borage oil or 1000-2000 mg of evening primrose oil per day	Reduces inflammation in the skin; improves moisture retention
Kindervital, by Flora Distributors (liquid multi-vitamin with minerals for children)	As directed	To ensure adequate nutrient support for children
Quercetin or grape seed extract	500 mg, three times per day	Anti-inflammatory; anti-allergy; halts histamine release
Digestive enzymes (Zymactive™)	1-2 capsules 15 minutes before every meal	Aids digestion; See HCl in Health Tips below

HEALTH TIPS TO ENHANCE HEALING

- Start a diet diary; write down everything that you eat to see if there is any correlation to symptoms. Ask for a referral to an allergy specialist and get tested for possible triggers. Some allergies may only be detected with the help of an ELISA (Enzyme-Linked Immunosorbent Assay)/ACT test. Once you know what you are allergic to, avoid those allergens.

- Have your thyroid checked. Low thyroid function impairs the immune system.
- Do not take immune boosters that enhance macrophage function as they will increase inflammation in the cells of the skin.
- Eat seven to ten half-cup servings of fruits and vegetables every day. If you haven't been eating raw veggies regularly, start with steamed; they will be easier on your digestive system. Eat plenty of cold-water fish (salmon, herring, halibut, mackerel), dandelion greens (available at health food stores or pick in areas not sprayed by pesticides) and essential fatty acid-rich seed and nut oils; these foods help heal eczema.
- Avoid deep-fried foods, meat, food that is high in sugar and other refined carbohydrates (like white bread), caffeine, alcohol and dairy products.
- If you suspect you have low stomach acid, take one capsule (600 mg) of hydrochloric acid (HCl) before a large meal. If symptoms worsen, stop – you do not have low stomach acid. If you feel the same or better, increase your dosage by one capsule at your next meal. Keep increasing the dosage up to a maximum of seven capsules or until you feel warmth in your stomach. If you feel the warmth, cut back to your dosage prior to having the feeling. Use fewer capsules for smaller meals.

OTHER RECOMMENDATIONS

- Use topical creams containing Celadrin or Herbacort (a combination of cortisone-like herbs) or chamomile cream (Camocare).
- Use hypoallergenic laundry detergents and rinse your bedding, towels and clothing twice to eliminate detergent residue. Do not use fabric softeners or dryer sheets; these are often a source of skin irritation and allergy.
- Drink water – 8 to 10 glasses of pure, clean, filtered water every day.

■ Long term use of cortisone ointments can cause serious side effects and skin thinning. They should not be used continuously. Avoid using them on small children, and determine underlying allergies quickly before chronic skin inflammation occurs.

Fibromyalgia (FM)

Almost 16 million North Americans suffer from fibromyalgia, a multisystem disorder. This common rheumatic syndrome has also been referred to as the "invisible illness" because of the difficulty in diagnosing it. The name fibromyalgia is rooted in Latin: "fibro," meaning supportive tissue; "myo," for muscle; and "algia" for pain. The hallmark of fibromyalgia is widespread pain throughout the muscles, stiffness and chronic aching. It affects women more than men, and usually strikes between the ages of 30 and 60 years. It accounts for 15 to 30 percent of all visits to rheumatologists. The pain of FM is thought to be caused by a tightening and thickening of the thin film of tissue that holds muscles together. A diagnosis of FM will be confirmed if your doctor finds pain or tenderness in 11 out of 18 trigger points located in the knees, hips, ribcage, shoulder and neck.

SYMPTOMS
Many of the symptoms of FM overlap with those of chronic fatigue syndrome (CFS). There is one main difference between the two: there is profound fatigue in CFS and profound muscle pain in FM. Treatments for CFS focus on eliminating viruses that may be causing the fatigue. FM treatments try to reduce inflammatory factors that cause the pain and swelling of joints and muscles. Due to the many symptoms of FM and CFS, a combination of therapies may be required to get the conditions under control.

The symptoms of FM are varied and no two sufferers are the same. They can include: allergies; anxiety; mental confusion; fatigue; dysmenorrhea; ridged fingernails; stiffness; inability to exercise; gastrointestinal problems; depression; mood swings; headaches; sensitivity to light, sound or odors; dizziness; heart palpitations; sleep disturbances; carpal tunnel syndrome; skin tender to the touch; swollen joints; total body aches and pain. Non-restorative sleep is a major symptom; those affected sleep, but never feel rested. When people describe their muscle fatigue, they liken it to shoveling snow or gardening for days without a break, or that the muscles are being stretched and torn.

The unique nature of the each person's collection of symptoms makes FM difficult to diagnose. Many tests, including urine, blood, CAT scan, magnetic resonance imaging, X-ray and more, may be conducted without any clear indication of what is wrong with the person. Sufferers are often referred to psychiatrists. Life becomes unbearable for those living with FM. It can also be difficult for family and friends to understand this shadowy disease.

CAUSES
No one cause can be pinpointed but it is believed that multiple stressors, a traumatic emotional or physical event and/or depressive episodes that upset the functioning of the immune system contribute to the disorder. It is suspected that a connection lies between FM and CFS since those with FM usually have a history of extreme, relentless fatigue. Viruses may have a hand in it, such as Epstein-Barr virus or fungus like *Candida albicans*. New research is showing that undetected Lyme disease may be the root cause. Heavy metal and chemical toxicity, as well as nutritional deficiencies, are major players in the progression of FM. Allergies are also thought to play a role in FM, and they must be diagnosed and eliminated to allow healing. Low sero-

tonin levels and low DHEA are also seen in those with FM. Physicians must peel away the causal layers of each symptom and treat each symptom individually in order to eliminate this disorder.

The Inflammation Factor

The immune cytokine Interleukin-6 is one factor that causes pain and inflammation. High levels of the stress hormone cortisol cause the immune system to secrete inflammatory factors, and high levels of cortisol also cause DHEA levels to drop. DHEA is an important anti-inflammatory hormone that reduces pain effectively. Many FM sufferers have found that none of the supplements they try work. There is a good reason for this. FM is made worse by the release of Interleukin-6, and unless we turn off this powerful inflammatory immune factor, we are not getting to the root of the problem.

PRESCRIPTION FOR HEALTH

Nutrient	Dosage	Action
Multivitamin with minerals	As directed	Provides a solid nutrient foundation that supports muscle, cartilage and bone development; helps support healthy immune function; controls inflammatory factors. Also aids the synthesis of collagen, the glue-like substance in cartilage, and reduces pain
Celadrin™	Orally: 1500 mg tablet/ capsule form or 1050 mg soft gel, per day Topical cream: apply twice each day	Reduces swelling and pain, and improves joint mobility; inhibits inflammation and joint destruction

Nutrient	Dosage	Action
Magnesium (either alone or in a combination of citrate, fumarate, glycinate, malate, succinate or aspartate)	200 mg, three times per day	Needed for 300 enzymatic reactions; calms inflammation in the muscles
Malic acid	1200-2000 mg per day	Detoxifies the body of aluminum and reduces pain of FM; works with magnesium
5-HTP	50-100 mg, three times per day	Increases serotonin levels; reduces anxiety and muscle pain; improves sleep and early morning stiffness; enhances mood; controls appetite
Valerian	As directed	Improves sleep; calms nerves
Melatonin	1-3 mg per night	Improves sleep
L-carnitine	500 mg per day	Improves energy production; eliminates fatigue

HEALTH TIPS TO ENHANCE HEALING

- Eat a balanced diet of fresh fruits and vegetables, healthy oils, nuts and seeds, whole grains and fresh wild fish to fight FM. Eat smaller meals more frequently throughout the day to maintain blood sugar levels.

- Avoid processed, refined foods; they are high in sugar, salt and hydrogenated fat.

- Drink plenty of pure, clean, filtered water – 8 to 10 glasses daily. For every cup of beverage (other than herbal tea) that you consume, drink another glass of water.

- Eliminate alcohol, smoking and caffeine.

- Get regular exercise, but don't overexert yourself. Gentle, moderate exercise improves your circulation and enhances your mood and overall well-being. Even walking to your mailbox or sitting in a chair and raising your arms and legs can be beneficial.

OTHER RECOMMENDATIONS

- Laugh! Rent videos, see a stand-up comic and hang around funny friends. Laughter as well as exercise can improve mood. Keep a positive frame of mind.
- Ensure adequate rest.
- Practise deep breathing exercises to ensure sufficient oxygen intake.
- Detoxification is extremely important. Saunas allow toxins to excrete from the skin; dry brushing before a shower or bath will increase circulation and stimulate lymph flow; and internal herbal cleanses combined with fiber will eliminate waste from the intestines and support the liver and kidneys. Have an Epsom salts and baking soda bath every night. Pour one cup of each into a bath; run the water through your shower filter rather than through the tap to ensure that you are not soaking in chlorinated water.
- Start a diet diary and write down everything you eat to see if there is any increase in symptoms or their intensity after you eat certain foods. Ask for a referral to an allergy specialist and get tested for possible triggers. Once you know what you are allergic to, avoid those allergens. Environmental allergies should be tested for as well.
- Have dental amalgams removed to reduce your toxic load.
- Massage, acupuncture and chiropractic treatments can help speed healing.
- When you are having a bad day, rest. On your good days, enjoy them to their fullest without overexerting yourself.
- Since there are multiple causes to this illness, there are multiple cures. What works for one person may not work for

another due to biochemical individuality. Do not give up; the most important gift is the power of faith.

Gingivitis

Gingivitis is a swelling or inflammation of the gum tissue. If gingivitis is not corrected, 30 percent of all cases will become periodontitis, a condition where the bacteria has spread from the gums to the bones, possibly resulting in lost teeth, an eroded jaw bone and dental surgery.

In the past gingivitis has not caused much concern, but a study conducted in 1998 found that compared to men with healthy gums, men with gum disease were four and a half times more likely to have heart disease. The connection is thought to come from the bacteria entering the bloodstream through the gums. Another study discovered that people with gum disease had 50 percent more plaque build-up in their carotid arteries than people with healthy gums. Plaque build-up is a major risk factor for stroke. In June 2000, it was announced that a study observing 1,000 pregnant women discovered premature deliveries were 8 times more likely if the patient had gum disease.

SYMPTOMS
The gums become bright red, tender, swollen, and will bleed readily. Gum tissue will withdraw from the teeth, leaving the patient with receding gums. Continual bad breath may also be present.

CAUSES
Bacteria that have not been removed by brushing and flossing sit under the gum line and eventually lead to infection. Other factors that can contribute to gingivitis are smoking, brushing

too hard, dental work that is too loose, nutritional deficiencies, stress, a weakened immune system and diets that are high in refined carbohydrates and sugar. Veterans who suffer from post-traumatic stress disorder have a higher rate of gum disease, including gingivitis.

Elevated hormones during pregnancy exaggerate the body's response to plaque in the mouth and increase the likelihood of getting gingivitis. If good oral hygiene is practiced, this should not become a problem. People with diabetes are known to be more prone to gingivitis than those without. However, when diabetes is well controlled, gingivitis is kept in check.

PRESCRIPTION FOR HEALTH

Nutrient	Dosage	Action
Multivitamin with minerals	As directed	Provides adequate nutrient support
Celadrin™	1500 mg tablet/capsule form or 1050 mg soft gel, per day	Inhibits inflammation
BB536 Bifidobacterium longum	As directed	Provides friendly, protective bacteria throughout the entire digestive system
Oil of oregano	3 drops, three times per day	Antibacterial; antifungal
Tea tree oil mouthwash	Gargle and swish twice daily	Antibacterial; antifungal
Goldenseal	20 drops per day	Antibacterial
CranMax™	1-2 capsules per day	May prevent bacteria from sticking to gums
Sage tea	Drink throughout the day	Soothes inflamed gums; antioxidant; anti-inflammatory

HEALTH TIPS TO ENHANCE HEALING

- Visit your dentist every six months to have hidden plaque removed from hard-to-reach areas.
- Chew gum with xylitol; it helps eliminate plaque and reduce gingivitis.
- Floss at least once every two days to remove plaque build-up under the gum line.
- When you brush your teeth, don't forget about your tongue. Either brush it or use a tongue scraper to remove the bacteria that are hiding in the mucus coating.
- Drink 8 to 10 glasses of clean, pure, filtered water daily – not from the tap. For every cup of juice, alcoholic or caffeinated beverage that you drink, add another glass of water.
- Eat a well-balanced diet that focuses on natural, whole foods such as whole grains, fresh fruits and vegetables, legumes, nuts and seeds and fresh fish. Avoid processed and refined foods that are high in sugar, white flour and bad fats.

OTHER RECOMMENDATIONS

- Stop smoking. Tobacco leaves a film of tar on the tongue, teeth and gums that can make infections worse and delay healing. It can also lead to oral cancer.
- If flossing is impossible to incorporate into your nightly routine, there is a toothbrush called Sonicare that emits acoustic energy. It cleans in areas once only reachable by flossing.
- When you can't brush, try fizzy tablets that have sodium bicarbonate, citric acid and silicon dioxide. They bubble up to remove leftover food particles. Or use a toothpick.
- Oral piercing increases the risk of infection so extra attention should be paid to oral hygiene.

Health Fact
Gingivitis was a common occurrence among soldiers during World War I and so it earned the nickname "Trench Mouth." The general belief was that it was caused by poor hygiene practices. While poor hygiene is a major cause, stress should not be overlooked as an important factor. Stress depresses the immune system and prevents it from reacting to the bacteria in a quick and efficient way.

Gout

Marked by an excruciatingly painful big toe, gout can also affect other joints. A common type of arthritis that affects mostly men – 95 percent of sufferers are male, gout arises when there is a build-up of uric acid in the body that crystallizes in the joints. Uric acid is a by-product of protein metabolism, especially from eating foods high in purines (including organ meats, beans and legumes) or drinking beer and wine. If there is too much uric acid in the blood, it is excreted to the joints, tissues, kidneys and tendons, where it causes inflammation. Gout comes and goes and its duration can vary from a few days to a few weeks, depending on how intense the causal factors were.

Pseudo-gout, officially known as calcium pyrophosphate dihydrate crystal deposition (CPPD), is similar to gout except that calcium crystallizes in the joints rather than uric acid. The presence of these calcium crystals weakens the cartilage, inducing it to break down more easily. The body reacts by creating inflammation to rid itself of the crystals.

SYMPTOMS

The uric acid crystals act as an abrasive, inducing pain and swelling. The initiating symptom of gout is a gnawing pain in the big toe, although it can strike the joints in the hand, wrist and knee as well. A fever or chills may accompany it. Walking can become difficult, as can sleeping if bedcovers rest on the toe. Pseudo-gout also causes redness, heat, pain and swelling in one or more joints. Left to progress, the cartilage can become so damaged that the bones rub together.

CAUSES

Gout has a genetic component and often runs in families. The most likely causes of gout are insufficient uricase (a digestive enzyme), too much protein and fatty food in the diet and excessive alcohol consumption. Stress is a trigger, as can be extra weight and a lack of exercise. Excess IL-6 is produced, causing inflammation and pain. The cause of pseudo-gout is unknown, but it is suspected that there is an abnormality in the connective tissue or cartilage, possibly a genetic factor.

High blood pressure and kidney disease are often present in those suffering with gout.

PRESCRIPTION FOR HEALTH

Nutrient	Dosage	Action
Multivitamin with minerals	As directed	Provides a solid nutrient foundation that supports muscle, cartilage and bone development; helps support healthy immune function; and controls inflammatory factors. Also aids the synthesis of collagen, the glue-like substance in cartilage, and reduces pain.

Celadrin™	Orally: 1500 mg tablet/ capsule form or 1050 mg soft gel, per day Topical cream: apply twice each day	Reduces swelling and pain, and improves joint mobility; inhibits inflammatory immune factors
Vitamin C	3000-5000 mg per day, in divided doses	Reduces serum uric acid
Quercetin	200-400 mg per day	Inhibits uric acid; anti-inflammatory
Magnesium	200 mg, three times per day	Especially important for pseudo-gout, where calcium is up-regulated
Fish oil (pharmaceutical grade)	3000 mg per day	Reduces inflammation; less stiffness in the joints
Zinc	15 mg per day	Remedies deficiency (common during gout attacks)
Enzymes (Zymactive™)	As directed. During gout attacks, use Zymactive three times per day on an empty stomach between meals	Potent anti-inflammatory when used between meals on an empty stomach

HEALTH TIPS TO ENHANCE HEALING

- Do not take niacin; it may promote a gout attack. Vitamin A in high doses is also not indicated for those with gout. Vitamin A can create toxicity due to the conversion to its more toxic form, retinoic acid, promoted by a dysfunction in enzymes found in those with gout.

- With pseudo-gout, it is important to have your iron levels checked to make sure that they are not too high (hemochromatosis). High iron levels are associated with pseudo-gout. If iron is high, give blood.

- Eating at least a half-pound of cherries or strawberries daily can neutralize uric acid. If they are out of season, cherry extract is available at health food stores – preferably organic and sugar-free.

- Eliminate organ and red meats, mushrooms, peanuts, meat-based gravies, shellfish, sardines, herring and mackerel from the diet during an episode of gout. Limited consumption may resume once symptoms are gone.
- Eat plenty of fresh fruits and vegetables (raw or as juices). Berries, onions and parsley are good sources of antioxidants. Drink at least 8 to 10 glasses of pure, clean, filtered water every day; it will help flush out the uric acid. For every cup of juice or caffeine beverage you drink, add another glass of water.
- Eliminate alcohol entirely. Beer is the worst beverage for promoting gout attacks.
- Restrict consumption of refined flour and simple sugars found in commercial bread, honey, fruit, juices and fructose.

OTHER RECOMMENDATIONS

- Avoid NSAIDs. See *Conventional Treatments* for information on the dangers of arthritis drugs.
- It is important for gout and pseudo-gout sufferers to get regular exercise, but if you are overweight, it is of even more benefit. Begin a moderate exercise program emphasizing the cardio component to help reduce weight, rather than embarking on a restrictive diet. Fasting or a sudden withdrawal of foods can increase uric acid.

Heart Disease

Heart disease is the category for about 30 cardiovascular conditions. The five main types are coronary artery disease (atherosclerosis or hardening of the arteries), heart muscle disease (cardiomyopathy), congestive heart failure (inability of the heart to pump enough blood), valve disorders (mitral valve prolapse) and arrhythmias (heartbeat rhythm irregularities). Heart disease is the leading cause of death in North America.

Women and Heart Disease

Heart disease is the number one killer of women of all ages each year. Women have finally achieved equality as they now have equal rates of heart disease to men, although more women than men die of heart attacks. Nearly one out of two women will die of cardiovascular disease. Women are also more likely than men to suffer a stroke after a heart attack. We have been taught that a heart attack is signalled by arm-clutching chest pain, but women can have very different heart attack symptoms to men. Unfortunately, many women are not aware that the risk is so great and do very little to protect themselves from the disease.

SYMPTOMS

Heart disease is a silent killer because people often do not know that they have it. New statistics published by the American Heart Association for 2004 show that 50 percent of men and 64 percent of women who died suddenly of heart disease during the course of their study had no previous symptoms. Be conscious of heart disease symptoms, including shortness of breath, irregular heartbeat, chest pain with exercise that subsides when you rest, or bouts of indigestion, a constricting feeling in your throat, profuse sweating for no apparent reason (not menopause). Seek emergency help for stomach pain, nausea and vomiting, dizziness, irregular pulse, light-headedness or unusual fatigue, and pain or numbness in the arms, back, neck or chest.

CAUSES

Until recently, heart disease was thought to be a problem solely caused by clogged arteries and high cholesterol. As noted earlier, half of all heart attacks occur in people with normal cholesterol and blood pressure (see page 10 for information on inflammation and heart disease). In fact, bacterial infections are also a cause of heart disease. Over a century ago, the medical establishment thought that heart disease was brought on by infections causing inflammation, but this theory was abandoned for what were new directions at the time. Now scientists have come full circle to focus on *chlamydia pneumoniae*. This bacterium is found in high concentrations in the blood of people who have had heart attacks. The infection theory is significant in that it points to the immune system and its failure to defend us from simple bacteria; by enhancing immunity, we may be able to prevent heart disease.

Although you may be predisposed to heart disease because of family history, this does not mean you must develop it. If you have a family history of coronary heart disease (CHD) you must be vigilant in making lifestyle choices that can prevent this deadly condition. Heart disease actually begins in the stomach. A poor diet of packaged or processed foods high in trans-fatty acids and devoid of fiber and nutrients (especially B vitamins and folic acid) are the main instigators of heart disease. Couple a poor diet with high stress, dehydration, aging, smoking, extra weight and a lack of exercise and sleep, and your risk climbs higher. Diabetes, high blood pressure or high levels of harmful LDL cholesterol or high blood homocysteine levels compound the problem. Homocysteine in the blood indicates a breakdown in chemical processes in the body and is strongly linked to heart disease. The risk of CHD is especially high for women of African-American descent.

PRESCRIPTION FOR HEALTH
If you are currently on Coumadin, high cholesterol or high blood pressure medication, talk to your physician or pharmacist about drug-nutrient interactions. Be aware that both high blood pressure and high cholesterol medications cause depletion of

coenzyme Q10, so you must supplement to ensure adequate levels. According to the *Drug-Induced Nutrient Depletion Handbook for Pharmacists*, if you are taking Lasix (flurosemide), you should be aware that Lasix depletes calcium; magnesium; potassium; vitamins B1, B6 and C and zinc. These nutrients must be replaced to prevent deficiency.

Nutrient	Dosage	Action
Multi-vitamin with minerals (without iron as high iron levels can increase risk of heart disease)	As directed on bottle	Provides adequate nutrient support
Celadrin™	1500 mg tablet/ capsule form or 1050 mg soft gel, per day	Inhibits inflammation; reduces CRP levels
Magnesium	200 mg, three times per day	Alleviates arrhythmia; essential for healthy heart muscle function
Vitamin B1	200 mg per day	Prevents depletion in those taking Lasix
Vitamin C (with bioflavonoids)	1000 mg, twice per day; bioflavonoids: 500 mg twice per day	Reduces symptoms and risk of heart disease; antioxidant; raises HDL (good) cholesterol; lowers blood pressure
Potassium	500 mg per day	Maintains healthy blood pressure
Vitamin E (with mixed tocopherols)	200-400 IU per day	Improves blood flow; reduces fatty plaques; supports immune function; acts as an antioxidant
Fish oil (pharmaceutical grade)	3000 mg per day	Reduces risk of heart disease; lowers triglycerides; anti-inflammatory

Nutrient	Dosage	Action
Coenzyme Q10	100-300 mg per day	Boosts energy production in the heart muscle; significantly improves heart function in those with congestive heart failure
Inositol hexanicotinate (non-flushing niacin)	500-1000 mg per day with meals. If you are not using non-flushing niacin, increase dosage slowly over three weeks until using 3000 mg per day, to avoid the harmless flushing of the skin	Lowers LDL cholesterol and triglycerides while raising HDL cholesterol. (Have liver enzymes and cholesterol checked every three months.)
Hawthorn extract (standardized 1.8% vitexin or 10% procyanidin content)	100-200 mg, three times per day	Double-blind studies show improvement in those with congestive heart failure
Pept Ace™	500 mg, three times per day	Significantly reduces blood pressure
Garlic Factors™	1-2 tablets per day	Improves circulation; reduces blood pressure
Gugulipid (standardized extract of mukul myrrh tree for 25 mg guggulsterone)	500 mg, three times per day	Increases liver's metabolism of LDL cholesterol to lower LDL cholesterol and triglyceride levels; raises HDL cholesterol levels; prevents atherosclerosis; reverses pre-existing plaque

HEALTH TIPS TO ENHANCE HEALING

■ Studies show that a diet emphasizing fresh fruits and vegetables, whole grains, legumes, lean meats and fish may lower risk of heart disease. Eating this way also provides valuable antioxidants, which are useful in combating chronic inflammation. Eat two eight-inch raw carrots per day, as this has been shown to reduce cholesterol by 50 points in a matter of weeks. Eat plenty of fresh-pressed garlic to lower blood pressure.

- The American Heart Association recommends two servings of fish per week to prevent heart disease. Fatty fish contains EPA and DHA, Omega-3 essential fatty acids. Alternatively, be sure to supplement with essential fatty acids to lower triglyceride levels and support normal cardiovascular health.

- Make sure that you stay hydrated with adequate amounts of clean, pure, filtered water to maintain blood flow. Studies show that drinking five glasses of water per day cuts your risk of stroke and heart attack in half.

- Reduce consumption of salt, caffeine and alcohol and be sure to get plenty of exercise followed by sufficient rest.

- Have your thyroid checked. Low levels of thyroid hormone cause heart palpitations in women and add to heart stress.

- Quit smoking and avoid second hand smoke.

- Insist that your doctor measure your homocysteine and C-reactive protein levels (both indicators of heart disease). Fortunately, high levels of homocysteine can be quickly addressed by supplementing with magnesium, B6, B12, folic acid and fish oils. High levels of C-reactive protein are reduced with Celadrin. See page 10 for more information on CRP.

- Studies show that holding on to anger is not only bad for your mood but is also linked to increased risk of heart disease.

- Many people with high blood pressure have the wrong ratio of potassium to salt. Reduce sodium intake by avoiding table salt and processed foods. Increase your intake of potassium-rich foods such as bananas, apricots, tomatoes, avocados, potatoes, lean chicken meat and fresh fish.

- Get adequate exercise. Walking 30 minutes three times a week cuts your risk of heart attack by about 30 percent. The more energetic your exercise, the greater your benefit: increasing your walking pace to two miles per hour or faster can reduce your risk up to 63 percent.

Inflammatory Bowel Disease, Irritable Bowel Syndrome, see *Bowel Disease*

Joint, Muscle and Tendon Injuries

Most of us have experienced a sprain or strain at some time during our lives. Injuries to muscles, tendons and joints are common. Maybe you slipped on an icy sidewalk, turned a screwdriver with too much force, or after months of inactivity, you started an exercise program and now feel stiff and sore all over. Exercise-induced injuries are adding to the accidental joint, muscle and tendon injury statistics. Baby boomers are participating in sports and exercise activities more than ever before. As a result, sports-related injuries for this group have increased by over 33 percent in the last decade. Health club memberships for people over the age of 55 have increased by 300 percent. Accordingly, injuries for this age group have skyrocketed. More than 10 million sports injuries are treated each year in North America.

SYMPTOMS

We know we have injured a joint, muscle or tendon because pain is the main symptom. There are many different types of injuries: sprains, strains, tendinitis, meniscal tears, osteochondritis dissicans, chondromalacia and bursitis, to name a few. Many components make up joints, protect the skeleton and ensure we have mobility. Muscles are bundles of fibers that contract. They are attached to bones. Tendons are tough bands of connective tissue that attach each end of a muscle to a bone. Ligaments surround joints and connect one bone to another. Bursas are fluid-filled sacs found at sites where friction occurs; they provide cushioning between structures. All of these components can become injured.

A *sprain* involves either a stretched or torn ligament, the elastic tissue that connects bones to one another. Symptom severity depends on the extent of the damage, and can include pain, a popping or snapping sound when the injury occurred, inflammation with pain, swelling and fluid build-up in the area and an inability to put weight on the affected limb. A *strain* is the result of a partial or completely torn muscle.

Tendinitis is an inflammation of a tendon, the fibrous cords that connect muscles to bones. Tendons of the hands are especially prone to inflammation. Trigger finger, where the finger tendon becomes inflamed and does not move as smoothly (often causing a popping sound), is a common type of tendinitis. The Achilles tendon in the heel and the tendons of the rotator cuff are also areas that can suffer tendinitis. Those with rheumatoid arthritis, scleroderma and gout can also develop inflammation in the sheaths that surround the tendons, causing extreme pain and lack of mobility.

Meniscal injury of the knee involves a tear to the meniscus. The knee pops when injured. It can be extremely painful and fluid may build up in and around the knee. A meniscal injury is often associated with a severe sprain.

Osteochondritis dessicans (OCD) happens when a bit of bone or cartilage weakens or breaks off from the end of the bone. OCD is common in teens whose bones are still growing. Symptoms include pain, swelling, stiffness, or a catching or popping sound in the joint.

Chondromalacia occurs when the cartilage in the knee softens. This can be caused by overuse (it is common in runners), injury or weak muscles supporting the knee. Pain when walking up hills or stairs is the main symptom of this condition.

Bursitis occurs when the bursa fills with excess fluid. Swelling, tenderness or pain are the main symptoms, and the area may be hot to the touch.

CAUSES

Overuse, injury, not warming up before exercise and repetitive activities are the most common causes of joint, muscle and tendon injuries. Diseases, including gout, arthritis and many autoimmune disorders, are also associated with inflammation and damage to these important structures.

PRESCRIPTION FOR HEALTH

Nutrient	Dosage	Action
Celadrin™	Orally: 1500 mg tablet/ capsule form or 1050 mg soft gel, per day Topical cream: Apply twice a day if skin is not broken	Reduces swelling and pain; improves joint mobility; is a potent anti-inflammatory
Multivitamins with minerals	As directed	To ensure adequate nutrient support
Arnica (homeopathic)	30c every 15 minutes for one to four hours after injury. Then take one dose every 24 hours until healed	Reduces pain and inflammation; speeds healing
Enzymes (Zymactive™)	1-2 tablets between meals on an empty stomach, three times per day	Reduces inflammation; speeds healing

HEALTH TIPS TO ENHANCE HEALING

- Do not apply heat or have a deep massage in the area of the injury for the first 24 hours after injury.
- Do not drink alcohol after an injury; it promotes bleeding and bruising and inhibits healing.

- A combination of rest, ice, compression and elevation known as R.I.C.E. therapy should be applied within 48 hours of the injury. Rest to ensure no further injury occurs; ice the area to ease pain and reduce swelling and inflammation; use compression to reduce swelling, bruising or bleeding; and elevate the injured area to further reduce swelling and move fluids away from the injured area. Make sure you elevate the injury above the level of your heart. Use pillows, lie down and rest.

- To prevent ice burns, never apply ice directly to the skin; wrap it in a damp towel. Apply for 20 minutes every 2 hours, until swelling is reduced. Do not apply ice if you have Raynaud's Phenomenon (see *Raynaud's Disease/Phenomenon* or *Scleroderma*).

- If the skin is not broken, use topical anti-inflammatory creams like Celadrin or homeopathic creams including arnica or Traumeel as directed.

- Stop repetitive activities. If you use a computer, ensure that the keyboard and mouse are at the correct height so as not to overextend muscles and ligaments.

OTHER RECOMMENDATIONS

- Drink 8 to 10 glasses of pure, clean, filtered water a day to ensure that joints and muscles are well-hydrated.

- Always perform stretching exercises before exercising to lengthen muscles so they contract more efficiently during exercise. Three to 10 minutes of slow exercise like walking or riding the stationary bike before working out will help protect you from injury.

- Take up yoga. It has been shown to be effective in reducing pain and inflammation

Lupus, *see Systemic Lupus Erythematosus*

Psoriasis

Psoriasis is a very common skin condition characterized by the rapid production of skin cells, leading to a congestion of cells on the skin's surface. The normal life cycle of skin cells is 28 days, but cells produced by psoriasis mature up to a thousand times faster than those of healthy skin. Psoriasis can also cause an inflammatory form of arthritis called psoriatic arthritis. More than 7 million North Americans have psoriasis, with its onset generally in the late twenties. According to The National Psoriasis Foundation, 56 million hours of productivity are lost annually in the U.S. due to psoriasis. Treatment costs US$1.6 to $3.2 billion every year.

SYMPTOMS
Raised patches of red with white flakes or scales appear on the torso, elbows, knees, legs, back, arms and scalp. When it is in the scalp, psoriasis can promote hair loss. In some people, the nails may become dull, pitted or ridged and may separate from the nail bed. Psoriasis fluctuates between periods of inflammation and remission and is categorized as mild, moderate or severe. If the skin becomes too badly damaged, there can be fluid loss, bacterial infection and an inability to regulate temperature. Approximately 400 people die every year from psoriasis. There are psychological ramifications to psoriasis as well, as people may feel shame, embarrassment, social rejection and anger due to a lack of understanding on the part of their peers. This psychological aspect can significantly affect relationships.

Arthritis similar to rheumatoid arthritis, called psoriatic arthritis, is sometimes present in those with psoriasis and it is very difficult to treat. There is pain, morning stiffness, swelling, reduced range of motion, pitting of the nails, tiredness and redness in the eye (conjunctivitis). In severe cases, it can lead to deformity of the joints and spine. Difficult to diagnose in people with subtle symptoms, it is believed that 10 to 30 percent of those with psoriasis will also develop psoriatic arthritis. It usually appears between 30 and 50 years of age.

CAUSES

The cause of psoriasis is unknown, but two theories have emerged: it is an autoimmune disorder, or it is caused by a bacterial "superantigen." Either way, there is a glitch in the immune system that tells the body to produce more skin cells. The immune system is often hyper-stimulated, promoting inflammatory cytokines in the skin cells. It may also be that the immune system, after a viral or bacterial infection, becomes primed to attack the skin.

Common triggers for psoriasis flare-ups are poor diet, incomplete protein digestion, a diet including excessive animal fat, bowel toxemia, impaired liver function, a superantigen or heavy alcohol consumption. Other triggers are reactions to medication, stress, sunburn, illness, injury, nerves or surgery.

PRESCRIPTION FOR HEALTH

Nutrient	Dosage	Action
Multivitamin with minerals	As directed	Provides adequate nutrient support
Celadrin™	Orally: 1500 mg tablet/ capsule form or 1050 mg soft gel, per day Topical cream: if skin is not broken, apply twice each day	Powerful anti-inflammatory; inhibits inflammation.
Fish oil (pharmaceutical grade)	3000 mg per day	Anti-inflammatory; promotes remission of psoriasis symptoms

Nutrient	Dosage	Action
High-lignan ground flax seeds	1-2 teaspoons per day	Improves bowel function; reduces bowel toxicity
Vitamin D	1000 IU per day	Reduces immune factors promoting inflammation of the skin
Milk thistle	100 mg, three times per day	Protects the liver; cleanses the blood
Comfrey or stinging nettle tea	Apply to head as a daily rinse	Loosens scales; heals scalp psoriasis

HEALTH TIPS TO ENHANCE HEALING

- See recommendations for *Arthritis* for those with psoriatic arthritis. Also see *Bowel Disease.*
- Avoid saturated fats; they promote flare-ups of psoriasis. Consume a diet that emphasizes natural, whole foods such as legumes, soy products, fresh fruit and vegetables, fish, healthy fats and oils, and nuts and seeds. Opt for foods high in vitamin E (cold-pressed oils, nuts, eggs, oatmeal, brown rice, corn meal, dry beans and green leafy vegetables) and vitamin C (onions, turnip greens, sweet peppers, currants, asparagus, Brussels sprouts). Avoid animal meat, choosing cold-water fish such as salmon, halibut and mackerel instead.
- Stress reduction is essential; 39 percent of those with psoriasis report stress initiates the disease.
- Eliminate caffeine, sugar and alcohol.
- Do not take immune boosters that enhance macrophages as this can cause inflammation in the skin.
- Improve digestion. Studies have noted that those with psoriasis have lower levels of hydrochloric acid. If you suspect you have low stomach acid, take one capsule (600 mg) of hydrochloric acid before a large meal. If symptoms worsen, stop – you do not have low stomach acid. If you feel the same

or better, increase your dosage by one at your next meal. Keep increasing dosage up to a maximum of seven capsules or until you feel warmth in your stomach. If you feel warmth, cut back to your dosage prior to the feeling. Use fewer capsules for smaller meals.

OTHER RECOMMENDATIONS

- Get a little sun. Psoriasis seems to abate during the summer months and that is thought to be a result of UV radiation.
- Allergies and food sensitivities are common for those with psoriasis. Start a diet diary and write down everything that you eat to see if there is any increase in symptoms or their intensity after you eat certain foods. Ask for a referral to an allergy specialist and get tested for possible triggers. Some allergies may only be detected with the help of an ELISA (Enzyme-Linked Immunosorbent Assay) test. Once you know what you are allergic to, avoid those allergens. Environmental allergies should be tested as well.
- Try natural alternatives to corticosteroid creams such as Celadrin cream or salves with capsaicin, licorice, chamomile and evening primrose oil. Botanical Therapeutics makes a great shampoo and conditioner for those with scalp psoriasis.
- Indulge in a sauna or steam bath.

Raynaud's Disease/Phenomenon

Raynaud's disease affects the circulatory system by constricting the arteries in the fingers and toes, causing them to spasm and causing the skin to discolor. The ears and nose may also be affected. It is more common in women, striking women nine times more often than men. Raynaud's disease usually begins in the early teens and becomes increasingly pronounced over the next thirty years. When the cause of the disease is known (such as autoimmunity, frostbite or surgical complications), it is called Raynaud's phenomenon.

SYMPTOMS

An attack is provoked by emotional stress or by exposure to cold (even touching something cold, such as a refrigerator door). The extremities tingle and, deprived of oxygen, turn white or blue. The loss of blood to the area for prolonged periods, often seen in scleroderma, can result in skin lesions, nail infections or tissue damage due to the lack of nutrients, so care must be taken to encourage blood flow. Gangrene is a rare result, but can occur.

CAUSES

Raynaud's disease is thought to be hereditary. Raynaud's phenomenon can be brought on by low thyroid, emotional stress, smoking, caffeine, nutritional deficiencies and drug reactions to beta blockers, decongestants, oral contraceptives and migraine relievers. Occupational environment or hazards such as working outdoors and exposure to chemicals such as vinyl chloride (PVCs) are also triggers. Those who use vibrating tools may find that Raynaud's is irreversible, persisting even after they no longer work with those tools. When Raynaud's is associated with lupus, rheumatoid arthritis, scleroderma or Sjogren's syndrome, the symptoms are much more severe.

PRESCRIPTION FOR HEALTH

Nutrient	Dosage	Action
Multivitamin with minerals	As directed	Reduces stress; improves metabolism and energy production; prevents nutrient deficiency

Celadrin™	Orally: 1500 mg tablet/ capsule form or 1050 mg soft gel, per day Topical: if skin is not broken, apply twice per day	Potent anti-inflammatory; controls immune factors that promote inflammation
Inositol hexaniacinate (non-flushing niacin)	1000 mg three times per day	Several human studies have shown fewer attacks after exposure to cold and enhanced circulation to fingers and toes
Vitamin E	400 IU twice daily	Promotes circulation
Magnesium	500 mg per day	Studies show reduction in reaction to cold
Evening primrose oil	3000 mg per day, in divided doses	Reduces reaction time to cold; reduces flare-ups
Fish oil (pharmaceutical grade)	3000 mg per day, in divided doses	Reduces flare-up and reaction to cold
Ginkgo biloba	120 mg per day	Improves circulation
Horse chestnut	As directed	Improves circulation

HEALTH TIPS TO ENHANCE HEALING

- Very important: eliminate caffeine from the diet – it constricts blood vessels.
- Stop smoking and avoid exposure to secondhand smoke. Nicotine constricts the blood vessels.

OTHER RECOMMENDATIONS

- Always dress warmly and avoid exposure to cold. Take warm footbaths or go to bed with warm leg wraps.
- Use Celadrin, borage or evening primrose oil as topical massage cream for your fingers and toes. Massage nightly for 2 to 3 minutes.
- Get plenty of rest and reduce stress. Keep a positive outlook. Practice deep breathing exercises, biofeedback, visualization and other therapies to calm the body.

- Regular exercise is beneficial for increasing circulation. Incorporate some new activities into your life; swing your arms regularly or rotate them backwards and forwards.
- It is very important to rule out food sensitivities. Start a diet diary and write down everything that you eat to see if there is any increase in symptoms, or their intensity, after eating certain foods. Ask for a referral to an allergy specialist and get tested for possible triggers. Some allergies may only be detected with the help of an ELISA (Enzyme-Linked Immunosorbent Assay) test. Once you know what you are allergic to, avoid those allergens. Environmental allergies should be tested as well.
- Have your physician test you for hypothyroidism.

Scleroderma

Systemic sclerosis, called scleroderma, is an autoimmune disease characterized by hardening and scarring of the skin. Chronic degeneration of connective tissue can also be seen in different organ systems, including the kidneys, lungs, heart and gastrointestinal systems. Scleroderma is highly individualistic, with the condition ranging from mild to severe to fatal. It is invisible when it affects the organs and very visible when it affects the skin. Four times as many women as men are affected, and it usually strikes after the age of 25. Young African American women are at high risk of developing scleroderma.

CREST syndrome is a mild skin sclerosis mainly limited to the fingers. It causes calcium deposits in the skin and throughout the body. Raynaud's disease, in which extremities such as fingers, toes, ears or nose turn white, is common. High blood pressure may also occur.

The immune system is dysfunctional in scleroderma. Autoantibodies and excessive immune activation by inflammatory cytokines, especially Interleukin-6 and Interleukin-1, are seen in scleroderma. Macrophages are also overactive.

SYMPTOMS

Initially the skin hardens and thickens; then it becomes tight, shiny and increasingly painful. The tissues calcify; the skin on the fingers and toes harden. It can affect large areas of skin or just the fingers. Difficulty swallowing and heartburn may be present, especially when the lower end of the esophagus is involved. The joints become stiff and achy. Fatigue, general weakness and weight loss are not uncommon, due to malabsorption caused by damage to the intestines. At some point, the skin becomes so hard the process stops and although movement may be somewhat restricted, it is not usually crippling. If, however, the disease affects the heart and kidneys, it can be fatal. Within the first seven years of a severe scleroderma diagnosis, seven out of ten patients will die.

CAUSES

Scleroderma results when there are spasms in the arteries supplying blood to the affected areas and there is abnormal collagen formation. Environmental factors are key in the development of scleroderma; this is evident by the fact that scleroderma-related antibodies are seen in the spouses of those affected with the disease. Ingestion of contaminated salad oils (rapeseed), as well as exposure to solvents like benzene, chemical compounds such as vinyl chloride (PVC) and silicone are primary triggers. Eosinophilia-myalgia syndrome (EMS), caused by ingesting contaminated L-tryptophan, resulted in scleroderma in many of those affected with EMS. Hand-arm vibration injury from using equipment like jackhammers can also cause scleroderma. An over-stimulated immune system is also clearly involved in scleroderma.

PRESCRIPTION FOR HEALTH

Recommendations below are focused on controlling the autoimmune process, increasing circulation to the skin and regulating collagen synthesis. If you also have Lupus, see *Systemic Lupus Erythematosus* for more information.

Nutrient	Dosage	Action
Multivitamin with minerals	As directed	Provides a solid nutrient foundation that supports muscle, cartilage and bone development; helps support healthy immune function; controls inflammatory factors. Also aids the synthesis of collagen (the glue-like substance in cartilage) and reduces pain.
Celadrin™	Orally: 1500 mg tablet/capsule form or 1050 mg soft gel, per day Topical cream: apply twice each day	Reduces swelling and pain; improves joint mobility; inhibits inflammation and joint destruction
PABA para-amino benzoic acid, (form used in studies was the potassium salt of PABA, called Potaba)	10 gm dosages per day were used in the research	Softens skin; increases skin mobility; increases survival rates. Do not take if you have vitilago.
Inositol hexaniacinate (non-flushing niacin)	1000 mg, three times per day	Reduces attacks after exposure to cold; enhances circulation to fingers and toes
Vitamin E	200-400 IU, twice per day	Promotes circulation
Magnesium	200 mg, three times per day	Potent anti-inflammatory
GLA from evening primrose oil (look for hexane-free) or borage oil	1000-2000 mg, three times per day	Reduces flare-ups; relieves pain
Fish oil (pharmaceutical grade)	3000 mg per day	Potent anti-inflammatory; important for cell membrane function

HEALTH TIPS TO ENHANCE HEALING

- Eliminate caffeine from the diet — it constricts blood vessels.
- Avoid animal meat; choose fish instead. Eliminate sugar and alcohol from the diet.
- Stop smoking and avoid exposure to secondhand smoke. Nicotine constricts the blood vessels.

OTHER RECOMMENDATIONS

- Rule out allergies. Start a diet diary and write down everything that you eat to see if there is any increase in symptoms or their intensity after you eat certain foods. Ask for a referral to an allergy specialist and get tested for possible triggers. Some allergies may only be detected with the help of an ELISA (Enzyme-Linked Immunosorbent Assay) test. Once you know what you are allergic to, avoid those allergens. Environmental allergies should be tested as well.
- Reduce stress.
- Rule out hydrochloric acid deficiency and take digestive enzymes.

Health Fact

A study was conducted to determine the effects of GLA on four patients who had had systemic sclerosis anywhere from 5 to 13 years. After one year of receiving 1 gram of GLA per day, all four felt relief from pain and saw improvement of skin texture, capillary walls and the healing of ulcers. In their conclusion, researchers suggested that 6 grams daily would be more beneficial.

Sjogren's Syndrome

Sjogren's (*show-grins*) syndrome is an autoimmune disorder or chronic inflammatory disease causing excessive dryness to the eyes and mucous membranes of the body. The immune system attacks the moisture-producing glands, causing infection, inflammation or corneal ulcers. It can appear as a primary condition or in conjunction with other autoimmune disorders such as rheumatoid arthritis and lupus. Two to four million Americans have Sjogren's syndrome. Nine out of ten people with Sjogren's syndrome will be female, predominantly aged forty to fifty.

SYMPTOMS

Primary Sjogren's syndrome is characterized by an inability of the eyes to tear. The eyes feel gritty and painful and are sensitive to light, smoke and fumes. Other areas that can be affected are the salivary glands, nose, skin and vagina. Mucous membranes lining the gastrointestinal tract and trachea can dry out and become painful, irritated and prone to infections. Pericarditis, or inflammation of the sac around the heart, can be a serious symptom of Sjogren's.

When Sjogren's syndrome is secondary to autoimmune disorders, dry mouth is significantly less present and symptoms expand to other areas of the body. There can be morning stiffness and pain in the muscles and joints, dry cough or other respiratory tract problems, nausea, indigestion and gastritis, renal disease, inflamed blood vessels, nerve problems (especially to the face), allergies and non-Hodgkins lymphoma. Fatigue can be debilitating.

The symptoms can range from mild to so severe they hinder quality of life. Some people may have a remission while others remain the same or become worse. Sjogren's can develop from a benign autoimmune disease into a lymphoid malignancy (non-Hodgkin's lymphomas, cancer).

CAUSES

Sjogren's is an autoimmune disease whereby the immune system destroys the exocrine glands (the fluid-secreting glands) and can advance to a systemic multi-organ attack. It is unknown what causes Sjogren's syndrome, but heredity may play a part, female hormones and viral infections are being investigated, in particular the retroviruses and herpes viruses (cytomegalovirus, hepatitis C, Epstein-Barr and herpes type-6). Triggers for Sjogren's syndrome include damage to the arteries or nerves in the face, food and environmental allergies, nutritional deficiencies, wearing contact lenses and smoking tobacco or marijuana.

PRESCRIPTION FOR HEALTH

Those with autoimmune disorders should not take immune boosters as they can over-stimulate B cell activity, promoting autoantibody production. Immune boosters, when taken long term, can enhance macrophage function and promote inflammatory cytokines. The German Commission E, a respected reference guide for herbs, does not recommend echinacea for those with autoimmune disease.

Nutrient	Dosage	Action
Multivitamin with minerals	As directed	Provides a solid nutrient foundation that supports muscle, cartilage and bone development; helps support healthy immune function; controls inflammatory factors. Also aids the synthesis of collagen (the glue-like substance in cartilage) and reduces pain.

Nutrient	Dosage	Action
Celadrin™	1500 mg tablet/capsule form or 1050 mg soft gel, per day	Powerful anti-inflammatory; inhibits inflammation
Bilberry	100 mg, twice per day	Improves circulation to the eyes
High-potency B-complex	2 capsules per day, with meals	Required for metabolism and immune function
Vitamin C	1000 mg, twice per day	Regulates immunity; combats stress
Vitamin E	100 IU per day	Reduces symptoms; improves tearing
Fish oil (pharmaceutical grade)	3000 mg per day	Anti-inflammatory; controls IL-1 and IL-6; increases the amount of tears
GLA from evening primrose oil or borage oil	1 gm, 3 times per day	Reduces recurrence and relapses; ensures proper function of Suppressor T-cells; anti-inflammatory

HEALTH TIPS TO ENHANCE HEALING

- Antihistamines and diuretics should never be taken by someone with Sjogren's syndrome.
- Stop smoking tobacco and marijuana and avoid exposure to secondhand smoke.
- Eliminate alcohol, sugar, salt and caffeine from the diet. They all contribute to dehydration.
- Suck on xylitol lozenges or chewing gum (sugar-free) to keep mucous membranes of the mouth moist.

OTHER RECOMMENDATIONS

- Rule out allergies. Start a diet diary and write down everything that you eat to see if there is any increase in symptoms or their intensity after you eat certain foods. Ask for a referral to an allergy specialist and get tested for possible triggers. Some allergies may only be detected with the help of an ELISA

(Enzyme-Linked Immunosorbent Assay) test. Once you know what you are allergic to, avoid those allergens. Environmental allergies should be tested as well.

- Weleda eyedrops, either Euphrasia D3 or Gencydo 1% or Cineraria Maritima D3 eyedrops, are extremely helpful for those with dry eyes.
- Reduce stress.
- Lack of saliva creates a vulnerability to bacterial infections in the mouth. Good personal and oral hygiene and preventative dental care should be practiced to minimize severity of symptoms. Get yourself an electric toothbrush and use it at least twice a day. Use mouthwashes that contain soothing herbs and aloe. Chew xylitol gum to prevent tooth decay and help moisturize the mouth.
- If vaginal dryness is a problem, use a water-based (not oil-based) lubricant.
- Avoid dry, windy climates, air-conditioning, dust and smoke. Keep your eyes moist with the help of a humidifier.
- If you have another autoimmune disorder, read that section as well for tips on how to alleviate those symptoms.

Sports Injuries, see *Joint, Muscle and Tendon Injuries*

Systemic Lupus Erythematosus

Systemic Lupus Erythematosus (SLE), commonly known as lupus, is a devastating form of arthritis. This is an autoimmune disease whereby the immune system attacks the connective tissue, affecting mostly the skin, joints, blood and kidneys. It may appear suddenly or develop over a number of years; most often it strikes children and women under the age of 40. In fact, women are afflicted 10 to 15 times more often than men are.

There are three types of lupus. Discoid lupus affects the skin only. Ten percent of those with discoid will develop systemic lupus, although it is believed that those people probably had systemic lupus with discoid lupus as an initial symptom. Systemic lupus involves the skin, joints and organs and is the type of lupus that is usually referred to when discussing lupus. The third type is drug-induced lupus.

Lupus is often a chronic condition with flare-ups and remission. For others, lupus is life-threatening when the lungs, kidneys or heart are attacked by antibodies.

SYMPTOMS
There are a number of markers for lupus. For discoid lupus, a rash on the neck or face and, in severe cases, symptoms of SLE may be present. SLE markers are a butterfly or discoid rash over the nose and cheeks like a mask; arthritic joint and muscle pain; mouth ulcers; sensitivity to light and worsening symptoms upon exposure to light; dry eyes and mouth; extreme fatigue; nervous system impairment; kidney damage detected by urinalysis; inflammation in the linings of the heart or lungs; low levels of red blood cells and specific white blood cells; and elevated levels of different antibodies.

People with lupus tend to be sensitive to sunlight, and their symptoms flare up and subside at varying intervals. A butterfly rash that appears across the nose is very common. Signs that a flare-up is going to occur include swollen glands and swollen, painful and inflamed joints. There can also be fever, headache, mouth ulcers, interstitial cystitis, weakness, hives, hair loss and weight loss. After an episode, scars on the skin may remain.

CAUSES

The actual cause of lupus is still unknown, however, researchers have discovered a variety of conditions that seem to contribute to it or provoke attacks. Viral or bacterial infections are leading suspects. Because women are the ones predominantly affected, it also suggests a link to excess estrogen or a deficiency in androgens (DHEA), both factors that trigger autoimmunity. Researchers are also studying ultraviolet radiation and its effect on clinical skin disease in lupus.

Other factors that are also commonly associated with a weak immune system and with lupus are stress, digestive problems due to weak stomach acid, fatigue, vaccination, food or environmental allergies (including toxic metal poisoning and hair dyes) and inherited predisposition.

Some drugs, including hydralazine, procainamide and beta-blockers, are responsible for creating what is known as drug-induced lupus (DIL); the condition will disappear upon withdrawal of medication.

PRESCRIPTION FOR HEALTH

Steroid medications including prednisone, immunosuppressive medications (including methotrexate and NSAIDs) are often used to control SLE. *Do not stop your medications. The following recommendations are to be used in conjunction with your medications.* After following this program for six weeks, have your physician test your auto-antibodies; your medication may need to be reduced. Auto-antibody levels should be checked again at the three-month and six-month point for further evaluation.

Nutrient	Dosage	Action
Multivitamin with minerals	As directed	Provides a solid nutrient foundation that supports muscle, cartilage and bone development; helps support healthy immune function; controls inflammatory factors. Also aids the synthesis of collagen (the glue-like substance in cartilage) and reduces pain.
Celadrin™	Orally: 1500 mg tablet/ capsule form or 1050 mg soft gel, per day Topical cream: apply twice each day	Reduces swelling and pain; improves joint mobility; inhibits inflammation and joint destruction
High-potency B-complex containing folic acid	2 capsules per day	Reduces stress; enhances metabolism; lowers homocysteine levels, thereby decreasing the risk of premature atherosclerosis
DHEA	200 mg per day; use under the guidance of your physician if your DHEA level is low	Reduces symptoms; may reduce the need for prednisone
BB536 Bifidobacterium longum	As directed	Improves intestinal flora to aid digestion
Fish oil (pharmaceutical grade)	3000 mg per day	Reduces or prevents pain and inflammation; can slow progression of autoimmune disease
Enzymes (Zymactive™)	1–2 capsules on an empty stomach between meals, three times per day	Acts as a potent anti-inflammatory; reduces pain

HEALTH TIPS TO ENHANCE HEALING

- Avoid alfalfa sprouts as they cause lupus flare-ups.
- Avoid the sun.
- Research has shown a diet low in bad fats (trans- and saturated

fats) and low in calories in general leads to a reduction in lupus symptoms and flare-ups. Patients experienced extended periods of remission.

- In order to maintain a higher quality of life, special attention must be paid to nutrition, supplements, exercise and positive thinking. Although there is an underlying genetic predisposition, avoiding and eliminating triggers can alleviate the severity and duration of symptoms and perhaps reduce the level of medication. Only 10 percent of those with lupus have a parent or sibling with it; only 5 percent of children born to those with lupus will develop it as well.

- Consume a diet that emphasizes natural, whole foods such as legumes, soy products, fresh fruit and vegetables, fish, healthy fats and oils to increase Omega-6 intake and nuts and seeds. Eat plenty of cold-water fish (halibut, herring, salmon, mackerel; canned sardines in olive oil are especially beneficial as they are high in Omega-3 EFA), which can keep inflammation down.

- Avoid caffeine, alcohol, dairy and animal products, processed foods containing sugar and additives, any vegetable in the nightshade family (white potatoes, peppers, eggplant, tomatoes).

- Stop smoking and avoid exposure to secondhand smoke. Nicotine constricts the blood vessels.

- Get plenty of rest and reduce stress. Keeping a positive outlook is essential. The Lupus Foundation of America offers much support in dealing with the illness. Practice deep breathing exercises, biofeedback, visualization and other therapies to calm the body.

- Regular exercise is beneficial for increasing circulation. Continue your exercise program if mobility is good, but not to the point where pain and inflammation flare up. Engage in activities (like water aerobics, swimming, cycling and yoga) that support body weight and cushion the joints from damaging impact.

OTHER RECOMMENDATIONS

- Have hair tested and analyzed for toxic levels of heavy metals present in the body.

- Start a diet diary; write down everything that you eat to see if there is any increase in symptoms or their intensity after eating certain foods. Ask for a referral to an allergy specialist and get tested for possible triggers. Some allergies may only be detected with the help of an ELISA (Enzyme-Linked Immunosorbent Assay) test. Once you know what you are allergic to, avoid those allergens. Environmental allergies should be tested as well.

- Consider having old mercury fillings removed and replaced with safer materials; however, ensure that you are not allergic to those substances before having them put into your mouth. If you choose to replace fillings, do it slowly over time so as not to release too much mercury into your bloodstream at once.

- When antigens and antibodies interlock, it is called an immune complex. Proteolytic enzyme therapy (Zymactive™) may help by penetrating the coating of the immune complex in the tissues and getting these factors into the bloodstream for elimination. This would stimulate the break-up of the immune complex and speed up the inflammation process to reduce tissue swelling. Due to the increased activity, it is acknowledged that the condition worsens for a short time before it gets better. Use this therapy with the supervision of a naturopath or physician.

- Avoid taking oral contraceptives, penicillin, hydraline, anti-convulsants, sulfa drugs and procaineamide. Ask your doctor if they are really necessary or if there are safer alternatives.

Resources

Ammon HP, Safayhi H, Mack T, Sabieraj J. "Mechanism of antiinflammatory actions of curcumine and boswellic acids." *J Ethnopharmacol*, 1993 Mar; 38(2-3):113-9.

Ammon HP. "Boswellic acids (components of frankincense) as the active principle in treatment of chronic inflammatory diseases." *Wien Med Wochenschr*, 2002; 152(15-16):373-8.

American Autoimmune Related Diseases Association, Inc. www.aardai.org

Aqel, MB. "Relaxant Effect of the Volatile Oil of Rosmarinus Officinalis on Tracheal Smooth Muscle." *Journal of Ethnopharmacology*, 1991; 33:57-62.

Arthritis Foundation, www.arthritis.org

Balasubramanyam M, Koteswari AA, Kumar RS, Monickaraj SF, Maheswari JU, Mohan V. "Curcumin-induced inhibition of cellular reactive oxygen species generation: novel therapeutic implications." *J Biosci*, 2003 Dec; 28(6):715-21.

Batmanghelidg, Fereydoon, *Your Body's Many Cries for Water*, Global Health Solutions, Inc., Falls Church, VA. 1997.

Bittiner SB, et al. "A Double-blind, Randomised, Placebo-controlled Trial of Fish Oil in Psoriasis." *The Lancet*, 1988; 1(8582):378-380.

Block, MT. "Vitamin E in the treatment of diseases of the skin." Clinical Medicine, January 1953; pp. 31-34 [in *Werbach*].

Bogaty P, Brophy J, Noel M, Boyer L, Simard S, Bertrand F, Dagenais GR. "Impact of Prolonged Cyclooxygenase-2 Inhibition on Inflammatory Markers and Endothelial Function in Patients With Ischemic Heart Disease and Raised C-Reactive Protein. A Randomized Placebo-Controlled Study." *Circulation*, 2004; Aug 9.

Bouic PJDB, et al. *The International Journal of Immunopharmacology*, Dec 1996; 18:(12):693-700.

Bouic, PJD. "Sterols/Sterolins, the natural, nontoxic immunomodulators and their role in the control of rheumatoid arthritis." *Arthritis Trust of America Newsletter*. Summer 1998.

Bradley, JD, et al. "Comparison of an Antiinflammatory. Dose of Ibuprofen, an Analgesic Dose of Ibuprofen, and Acetaminophen in the Treatment of Patients with Osteoarthritis of the Knee." *The New England Journal of Medicine*, 1991; 325:87-91.

Broadhurst, C Leigh. *Natural Relief from Asthma*. Alive Books, Burnaby, BC. 2000.

Broughton, KS, et al. "Reduced Asthma Symptoms with n-3 Fatty Acid Ingestion Are Related to 5-series Leukotriene production." *American Journal of Clinical Nutrition*, 1997; 65:1011-17.

Burt CW, Overpeck MD. "Emergency visits for sports-related injuries." *Ann Emerg Med*, March 2001; 37:301-308.

Butland BK, Fehily AM, and Elwood PC. "Diet, lung function, and lung function decline in a cohort of 2512 middle-aged men." *Thorax*, 2000; 55:102-108.

Burns AJ, Rowland IR. "Anti-carcinogenicity of probiotics and prebiotics." *Curr Issues Intest Microbiol*, 2000 Mar; 1(1):13-24. Review.

Callahan, LF, Rao J, Boutaugh M. "Arthritis and Women's Health: Prevalence, Impact and Prevention." *Am J Pre Med*, 1996; 12(5):401-409.

Carey IM, DP Strachan, DG Cook. "Effects of changes in fresh fruit consumption on ventilatory function in healthy British adults." Am J *Respir Crit* Care Med, 1998; 158:728-733.

Carson-DeWitt, RS. "Systemic lupus erythematosus." *Gale Encyclopedia of Medicine*, Gale Research Group, 1999.

Caughey DE, Grigor RR, Caughey EB, et al. "*Perna canaliculus* in the treatment of rheumatoid arthritis." *Eur J Rheumatol Inflamm*, 1983; 6:197-200.

Celadrin, www.celadrin.com

Childs, Nathan D. "Could Lyme Vaccine Trigger Autoimmune Arthritis?" *Pediatric News*, 1999; Volume 33, 6:20.

Cohen, HA, et al. "Blocking Effect of Vitamin C in Exercise Induced Asthma." *Archives of Pediatric Adolescent Medicine*, 1997; 151:367-70.

Crohn's and Colitis Foundation of America, www.ccfa.org

Conway B, Rene A. "Obesity as a disease: no lightweight matter." *Obes Rev*, 2004 Aug; 5(3):145-51.

Custovic A, Simpson A, Chapman MD, Woodcock A. "Allergen avoidance in the treatment of asthma and atopic disorders." *Thorax*, 1998; 53:63-72.

D'Ambrosio, E, et al. "Glucosamine Sulfate: A Controlled Clinical Investigation in Arthrosis." *Pharmatherapeutica*, 1981; 2(8):504 –510.

De Caterina R, Liao JK, Libby P. "Fatty acid modulation of endothelial activation." *Am J Clin Nutr*, 2000; 213s-23s.

Delport, R. et al. "Vitamin B6 Nutritional Status in asthma: The Effect of Theophylline therapy on Plasma Pyridoxal-5-Phosphate and Pyridoxal Levels." Int J Vitam Nutr Res, 1988; 58(1):67-72.

Deodhar SD, et al. "Preliminary studies on anti-rheumatic activity of curcumin." Ind J Med Res, 1980; 71:633.

Dew MJ, Evans BK, Rhodes J. "Peppermint oil for irritable bowel syndrome: a multicentre trial." British Journal of Clinical Practice. 1984, 38:394-8.

Dexter P., and Brandt, K. "Distribution and Predictors of Depressive Symptoms of Osteoarthritis." The Journal of Rheumatology, 1994; 21(2): 279-286.

Dixon, J, et al. Second-line Agents in the Treatment of Rheumatic Diseases. New York, Marcel Dekker, 1992.

Droste JHJ, et al. "Does the use of antibiotics in early childhood increase the risk of asthma and allergic disease?" Clinical and Experimental Allergy, 2000; 30:1547-1553.

Emelyanov A, Fedoseev G, Krasnoschekova O, et al. "Treatment of asthma with lipid extract of New Zealand green-lipped mussel: a randomised clinical trial." Eur Respir J, 2002; 20:596–600.

Fabender, HM, et al. "Glucosamine sulfate compared to ibuprofen in osteoarthritis of the knee." Osteoarthritis and Cartilage, 1994; 2(1):61-69.

Finnegan, John, The Facts About Fats. Celestial Arts, 1993.

Fujita H, Yasumoto R, Hasegawa M, Ohshima K. "Antihypertensive activity of 'Katsuobushi Oligopeptide' in hypertensive and borderline hypertensive subjects." Jpn Pharmacol Ther, 1997; 25:147-51.

Fujita H, Yamagami T, Ohshima K. "Effect of an ace-inhibitory agent, katuobishi oligopeptide, in the spontaneously hypertensive rat and in borderline and mildly hypertensive subjects." *Nutr Res*, 2001; 21:1149-58.

Galland, L. "Increased Requirements for Essential Fatty Acids in Atopic Individuals, A Review with Clinical Descriptions." *American Journal of Clinical Nutrition*, 1986; 5:213-228.

Gay, G. "Another Side Effect of NSAIDs." *Journal of the American Medical Association*, 1990; 264(20):2677-2678.

Gecht, MR, et al. "A Survey of Exercise Beliefs and Exercise Habits Among People with Arthritis." *Arthritis Care and Research*, 1996; 9(2):82-88.

Gemmell E, Carter CL, Seymour GJ. "Mast cells in human periodontal disease." *J Dent Res*, 2004 May; 83(5):384-7.

Genco, R, et al. "Periodontal disease and risk for myocardial infarction and cardiovascular disease." *CVR&R*, March 1998; pp. 34-40.

Germano, Carl, and Cabot, William, *Nature's Pain Killers*. Kensington Books, New York, NY.

Geusens P, et al. "Long-term effect of omega-3 fatty acid supplementation in active rheumatoid arthritis. A 12-month, double-blind, controlled study." *Arthritis Rheum*, 1994; 37(6): 824-829.

Gibson RG, Gibson SL. "Green-lipped mussel extract in arthritis." *The Lancet*, 1981; 1:439 [letter].

Gibson SLM, Gibson RG. "The treatment of arthritis with a lipid extract of Perna canaliculus: a randomized trial." *Comp Ther Med*, 1998; 6:122-6.

Grant IR, Ball HJ, Rowe MT. "Inactivation of Mycobacterium paratuberculosis in cow's milk at pasteurization temperatures." *Applied and Environmental Microbiology*, 1996; 62:631-636.

Grave, G. "Antioxidant Nutrients in Inflammatory Bowel Disease." *Crohn's & Colitis Foundation of America physician letter.* www.ccfa.org

Grimble RF, Tappia PS. "Modulation of pro-inflammatory cytokine biology by unsaturated fatty acids." *Z Ernahrungswiss*, 1998; 7-65.

Gupta, MB, et al. "Anti-inflammatory and Antipyretic Activities of B-sitosterol." *Planta Medica*, 1980; 339:157-163.

Gursel T, Firat S, Ercan ZS. "Increased serum leukotriene B4 level in the active stage of Rheumatoid arthritis in children." *Prostaglandins Leukot Essent Fatty Acids*, 1997; 56:205-207.

Harries AD, and Heatley RV. "Nutritional disturbances in Crohn's disease." *Postgraduate Medical Journal*, 1983; 50:690-7.

Hay, Louise L, *Heal Your Body*. Hay House, Santa Monica, CA 1988

Henderson WR Jr. "The role of leukotrienes in inflammation." *Ann Intern Med*, 1994; 121:684-97.

Hermon-Taylor, John, Nick Barnes, Chris Clarke and Caroline Finalyson, "Mycobacterium paratuberculosis Cervical Lymphadenitis followed five years later by terminal ileitis similar to Crohn's Disease." *British Medical Journal*, February 7, 1998.

Hertog, ML and Hollman, PH. "Potential Health Effects of the Dietary Flavonol Quercetin." *European Journal of Clinical Nutrition*, 1996; 50:63-71.

Hesslink R Jr, Armstrong D 3rd, Nagendran MV, Sreevatsan S, Barathur R. "Cetylated fatty acids improve knee function in patients with osteoarthritis." *J Rheumatol*, 2002 Aug; 29(8):1708-12.

Hodge L, Salome CM, Peat JK, et al. "Consumption of oily fish and childhood asthma risk." *Medical Journal of Australia*, 1996; 164:137-40.

Hodgkinson, R and Woolf, D. "A Five Year Clinical Trial of Indomethacin in Osteoarthritis of the Hip Joint." *ACTA Orhtop Scand*, 1979; 50:169 -170.

Host, A. "Cow's Milk Allergy." *Journal of the Royal Society of Medicine*, 1997; 90:34-39 supplement.

Isolauri, F, et al. "Breast feeding of Allergic Infants." *Pediatrics*, 1999; 134:27-32.

Izaka, K, et al. "Gastrointestinal absorption and anti-inflammatory effect of bromelain." *Jpn J Pharmacol*, 1972; 22:519.

Jacob, SW, Lawrence, RM, Zucker, M. *The Miracle of MSM: The Natural Solution for Pain*. Penguin Putnam, Inc., New York, NY. 1999.

Jefferies, WM. "Cortisol and Immunity." *Medical Hypotheses*, 1991; 34:203.

Jensen, MN. "Good health requires good gums." *Science News*, May 9, 1998; 153:300-1.

Kitts, D. et al. "Adverse Reactions to Food Constituents: Allergy Intolerance and Autoimmunity." *Canadian Journal of Physiology and Pharmacology*, 1997; 75:241-254.

Kraemer WJ, Ratamess NA, Anderson JM, Maresh CM, Tiberio DP, Joyce ME, Messinger BN, French DN, Rubin MR, Gomez AL, Volek JS, Hesslink R Jr. "Effect of a cetylated fatty acid topical cream on functional mobility and quality of life of patients with osteoarthritis." *J Rheumatol*, 2004 Apr; 31(4):767-74.

Kuvaeva I, et al. "The microecology of the gastrointestinal tract and the immunological status under food allergy." *Nahrung*, 1984; 28:689-93. In *Nutritional Influences on Illness*, Werbach, Keats Publishing Corp, New York, NY, 1987.

Langer, Stephen, MD and James F. Scheer. *Pocket Guide to Natural Health*. Twin Stream, Keats Publishing Corp, New York, NY, 2001.

Li M, Yang B, Yu H, Zhang H. "Clinical observation of the therapeutic effect of ginkgo leaf concentrated oral liquor on bronchial asthma." *CJIM*,1997; 3:264–67.

Lichtenstein, LM. "Allergy and the Immune System." *Scientific America*, 1993; Sept:116-124.

Linos A, Kaklamani VG, Kaklamani E, et al. "Dietary factors in relation to rheumatoid arthritis: a role for olive oil and cooked vegetables?" *Am J Clin Nutr*, 1999; 1077-82.

Lowe GD, Rumley A, McMahon AD, Ford I, O'Reilly DS, Packard CJ. "West of Scotland Coronary Prevention Study Group. Interleukin-6, fibrin D-dimer, and coagulation factors VII and XIIa in prediction of coronary heart disease." *Arterioscler Thromb Vasc Biol*, 2004 Aug; 24(8):1529-34.

Lupus Foundation of America, www.lupus.org

Mastrandrea F, Coradduzza G, Serio G, Minardi A, Manelli M, Ardito S, Muratore L. "Probiotics reduce the CD34+ hemopoietic precursor cell increased traffic in allergic subjects." *Allerg Immunol* (Paris), 2004 Apr; 36(4):118-22.

Matricardi PM, et al. "Exposure to food-borne and orofecal microbes versus airborne viruses in relation to atopy and allergic asthma: epidemiological study." British Medical Journal, 2000; 320:412-7.

Matsumoto S, Watanabe N, Imaoka A, Okabe Y. "Preventive effects Bifidobacterium- and Lactobacillus-fermented milk on the development of inflammatory bowel disease in senescence-accelerated mouse P1/Yit strain mice." Digestion, 2001; 64(2):92-9.

McNeal, RL. "Aquatic Therapy for Patients with Rheumatic Disease." Rheumatic Disease Clinics of North America, 1990; 16(4):915-943.

Mittman, P. "Randomized double-blind study of freeze-dried Urtica dioica in the treatment of allergic rhinitis." Planta Med, 1990; 56:44-7.

Morreale, P, et al. "Comparison of the anti-inflammatory efficacy of chondroitin sulfate and diclofenac sodium in patients with knee osteoarthritis." J Rheumatol, 1996; 23(8):1285-1391.

Moreland, LW. "Treatment of Rheumatoid Arthritis with Recombinant Human Tumor Necrosis Factor Receptor (p75) Fc fusion." New England Journal of Medicine, 1997; 337(3):141-7.

Murray, MT. Encyclopedia of Nutritional Supplements. Prima Publishing, Rocklin, CA. 1996.

Murray, MT. Arthritis: How You Can Benefit from Diet, Vitamins, Minerals, Herbs, Exercise and Other Natural Methods. Prima Publishing, CA. 1994.

Morreale, P, et al. "Comparison of the anti-inflammatory efficacy of chondroitin sulfate and diclofenac sodium in patients with knee osteoarthritis." J Rheumatol, 1996; 23(8):1285-1391.

Nanda R, et al. "Food intolerance and irritable bowel syndrome." *Gut*, 198; 30(8):1099-1104.

National Psoriasis Foundation, www.psoriasis.org

Newman, NM, et al. "Acetabular Bone Destruction Related to Nonsteroidal Antiinflammatory Drugs." *The Lancet*, 1985; 2:11-14.

Newmark, Thomas M and Paul Schlulick. *Beyond Aspirin*. Hohm Press, Prescott, AZ. 2000.

Neuman I, Nahum H, Ben-Amotz A. "Reduction of exercise-induced asthma oxidative stress by lycopene a natural antioxidant." *Allergy*, 2000; 55:1184-1189.

Nossal, GJV. "Immunological Tolerance: Collaboration Between Antigen and Lymphokines." *Science*, 1989; 245:147-153.

Older SA, Battafarano DF, Enzenauer RJ, Krieg AM. "Can immunization precipitate connective tissue disease? Report of five cases of systemic lupus erythematosus and review of the literature." *Semin Arthritis Rheum*, 1999 December; 29(3): 131-9.

Pavlidis, NA, Karsh J, Moutsopoulos HM. "The clinical picture of primary Sjogren's syndrome: A retrospective study." *J Rheumatology*, 1982; 9:685-690.

Perneger, TV, et al. "Risk of Kidney Failure Associated with the Use of Acetaminophen, Aspirin, and Nonsteroidal Anitiinflammatory Drugs." *New England Journal of Medicine* 1994; 331(25):1675-1679.

Petri, Michelle, et al. "Plasma homocysteine as a risk factor for atherothrombotic events in systemic lupus erythematosus." *The Lancet*, October 26, 1996; 348:1120-24.

Pinget M, Lecomte A. "The effects of harpagophytum capsules in degenerative rheumatology." *J Medecine Actuelle*, 1985; 12(4): 65-7.

Pipitone, VR. "Chondroprotection with Chondroitin Sulfate." *Drugs in Experimental and Clinical Research*, 1991; 17(1):3-7.

Rennie, J. "The Body Against Itself." *Scientific American*, December 1990; 76-85.

Ridker PM. "High-sensitivity C-reactive protein, inflammation, and cardiovascular risk: from concept to clinical practice to clinical benefit." *Am Heart J*, 2004 Jul; 148 (1 Suppl):S19-26.

Rose, NR, Mackay IR, ed., *The Autoimmune Diseases*. Academic Press, San Diego, CA, 1998.

Ruiz-Gutierrez V, Muriana FJ, Guerrero A, et al. "Plasma lipids, erythrrocyte membrane lipids and blood pressure of hypertensive women after ingestion of dietary oleic acid from two different sources." *J Hypertens*, 1996; 483-90.

Samuel, MP, et al. "Fast Food Arthritis, a Clinic Pathologic Study of Post-salmonella Reactive Arthritis." *Journal of Rheumatology*, 1995; 22:1947-52.

Sata N, Hamada N, Horinouchi T, Amitani S, Yamashita T, Moriyama Y, Miyahara K. "C-reactive protein and atrial fibrillation. Is inflammation a consequence or a cause of atrial fibrillation?" *Jpn Heart J*, 2004 May; 45(3):441-5.

Schmid, et al. "Analgesic effects of willow bark extract in osteoarthritis: results of a clinical double-blind trial." *Fact*, 1998; 3:186.

Schwartz, ER. "The modulation of osteoarthritis development by Vitamin C and Vitamin E." *Int J Vit Nutr Res*, 1984; 26:141.

Scleroderma Foundation, www.scleroderma.org

Shahani, et al. "Benefits of Yogurt." *International Journal of Immunotherapy*, 1993; 9(1)65-68.

Sheldon, T. "Link between pollution and asthma uncovered." *British Medical Journal*, March 20, 1999. www.bmj.com

Shoda A, et al. "Therapeutic efficacy of N-2 polyunsaturated fatty acid in experimental Crohn's disease." *Journal of Gasteroenterology*, 1995; 30:(sup 8) 98-101.

Singh GB, Atal CK. "Pharmacology of an extract of salai guggal ex-Bosewellia serrata, a new non-steroidal anti-inflammatory agent." *Agents Action*, 1986; 18:407-12.

Sjogren's Syndrome Foundation, Inc., www.sjogrens.com

Strong, AMM, et al., "The effect of oral linoleic acid and gamma-linolenic acid (Efamol)." *British Journal of Clinical Practice*, November/December 1985, p. 444 [in Werbach].

Theodosakis, J. *The Arthritis Cure, New Hope For Beating Arthritis*, St. Martin's Press, New York 1997.

Traut, EF, Thrift, CB. "Obesity in Arthritis: Related Factors, Dietary Factors." *Journal of the American Geriatric Society*. 1969; 17:710-717.

Van Vollenhoven, RF, et al. "An open study of dehydroepiandrosterone in systemic lupus erythematosus." *Arthritis and Rheumatism*, 1994; 37:1305-10.

Vaz, AL. "Double-blind Clinical Evaluation of the Relative Efficacy of Ibuprofen and Glucosamine Sulphate in the Management of Osteoarthrosis of the Knee in Out-patients." *Current Medical Research and Opinion*, 1982; 8(3):145-149.

Voelker, R. "Ames Agrees with Mom' Advice: Eat Your Fruits and Vegetables." *The Journal of the American Medical Association*, 1995; 273(14):1077-1078.

Werbach, Melvyn R, MD. *Healing Through Nutrition*. HarperCollins Publishers, New York, NY. 1993.

Werbach, Melvyn R, MD. *Nutritional Influences on Illness. A Sourcebook of Clinical Research*, 2nd ed., Third Line Press, Tarzana, CA, 1990.

Whitaker, Julian. "Research Roundup: Mustaches." *Healthy & Healing*, February, 2001; 11(2).

Whitaker, Julian. "What to Add to Your Multivitamin to Address Specific Health Conditions." *The Whitaker Wellness Program: Part 3*. Phillips Publishing, Inc. Potomac, MD. 1999.

Whitaker, Julian. "Research Roundup: Cranberries." *Health & Healing*, December 2000; 10(12).

Whitaker, Julian. "Save Your Teeth and Your Health." *Health & Healing*, August 2000; 10(8).

Whitaker, Julian. "Research Roundup: Supplements." *Health & Healing*, January 2001; (11)1.

Whitehouse MW, Marcides TA, Kalafatis N, et al. "Anti-inflammatory activity of a lipid fraction (lyprinol) from the NZ green lipped muscle." *Inflam Pharmacol*, 1997; 5:237-46.

Wilson PW. "Assessing coronary heart disease risk with traditional and novel risk factors." *Clin Cardiol*, 2004 Jun; 27(6 Suppl 3):1117-11.

Yamamoto M, et al. "Anti-inflammatory Active Constituents of Aloe arborescens Miller." Agric. Biol. *Chem*, 1991; 55(6):1627-1629.

Yoshimoto, T, et al. "Flavonoids: Potent Inhibitors of Arachidonate-5-lipoxygenase." *Biochemical Biophysiolgical Research Communication*, 1983; 116:612-618.

Ziboh, VA, et al. *Arch Dermatol*, November 1986.

Also by Lorna R. Vanderhaeghe, BSc

The Immune System Cure:
Nature's Way to Super-Powered Health
with Patrick JD Bouic, PhD

Healthy Immunity:
Scientifically Proven Natural Treatments for Conditions from A-Z

Healthy Fats for Life:
Preventing and Treating Common Health Problems with
Essential Fatty Acids with Karlene Karst, BSc, RD.

No More HRT:
Menopause Treat the Cause with Dr. Karen Jensen

An A-Z Woman's Guide to Vibrant Health: Prevent and Treat the
Top 25 Female Health Conditions

The Body Sense Natural Diet Program: Six Weeks to a Slimmer,
Healthier You

For more information about Lorna Vanderhaeghe,
visit www.healthyimmunity.com